ENERGIZE

A Guide to Revitalizing Body, Mind, and Spirit using
Ancient and Modern Techniques via

Dynamic Self-Love

By

Robert Selman, Ph.D.

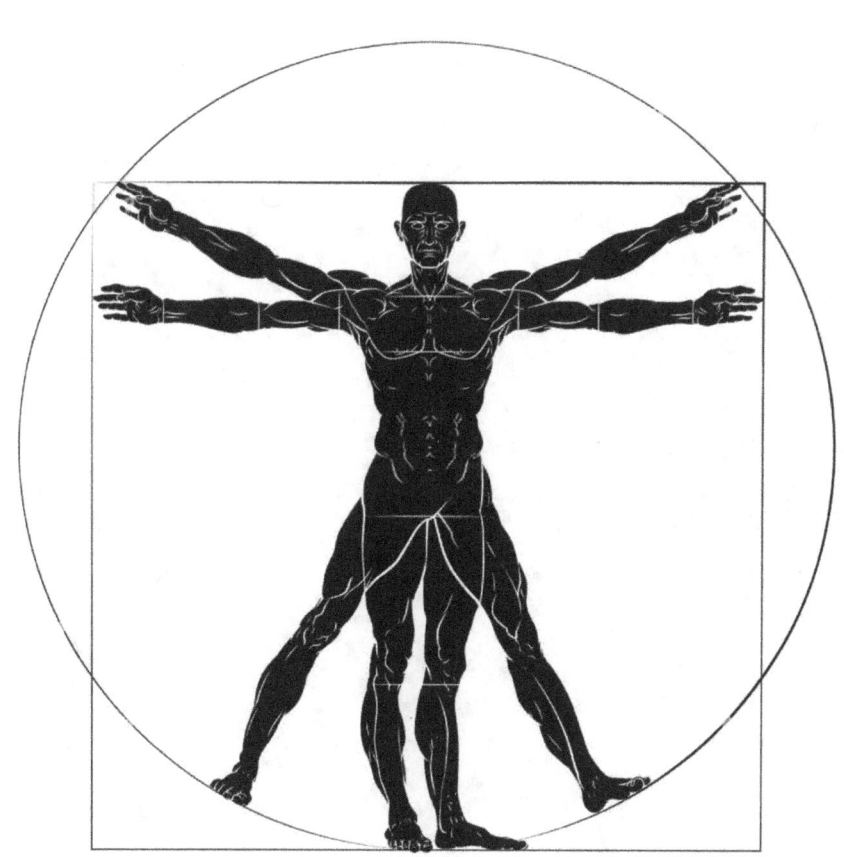

www.robertselman.com

Manufactured in the United States of America
ISBN: 978-1-312-06601-4

—Part 1—
Body

-Foreward-

When I was 20 years old, I attended college in Monterey, California. I borrowed my roommate's 650 BSA motorcycle to pick up a friend for an evening ride in her neighborhood. As we road along her street, we passed an area where the street lamps were still in the process of installation. The road went dark, and I could only see the white line in the middle of the road reflected by the single headlight beam. Suddenly, the white line disappeared, and I saw dirt instead of the blacktop road.

All went black. The life I knew had come to an end. Suddenly, the people I loved flashed in front of my eyes. Sparked was a vision of my mom and dad, my two sisters, my grandmother and grandfather, and finally, my girlfriend. Once again, all went black a second time. I then noticed an ever-so-slight sensation beginning to grow in my solar plexus. It was a light vibration of white energy expanding in all three dimensions, commencing from the area of my core abdomen. This vibration of white energy grew more prominent and robust, finally replacing the sense of my body with a stronger, more vivid, electrifying sense of existence. This transformation grew and replaced the experience of where my body had once been. I was now a hovering, egg-shaped field of white vibratory energy and began sensing movement.

I started moving up and to the left. I could sense an enormous source of white energy in the distance, and I had a sense I was traveling to meld and blend with this more expansive white light. In the distance, I could hear my friend shaking my body, then walking away, saying, "I'm going to die, I'm going to die." As I began melding with that more incredible white energy source, a male voice said, "You had a motorcycle accident. Your friend is hurt. You have to go back and help."

Just as I traveled up and to the left, I sensed movement going down and to the right until I found myself back in my body. I called out and felt a terrible pain in my stomach. Suddenly, this pain subsided, and I stood up and walked over to her, stating, "You're not going to die." I beckoned her to lie down and held her head on my lap. I again felt pain in my stomach, so I placed her head on the ground. From a distance, I saw the headlights of an oncoming car. I stood in front of the headlights and waved both arms to signal the driver to stop. As the car drew near, the passenger window opened. I talked to a man, saying, "We had a motorcycle accident. We need help."

The man stepped out of the car while the driver, his wife, went to fetch help. I told this man I had to lie down and did so. I could feel my breathing growing more and more restricted, struggling to get enough air into my lungs. Shortly after, an ambulance arrived, taking my friend and me to the hospital.

While lying in the ambulance, my entire body was unavailable, and I couldn't even move my eyes. I gazed at the wooden panels of the headliner in the ambulance and fought with sheer willpower to breathe. I found as time passed, my breathing grew shallower and more restrictive. However, I needed air and used every ounce of strength to force air into my lungs. This experience focused my attention solely to concentrate on inhaling air. With every inhalation, the difficulty of taking the next breath increased.

Finally, we reached the hospital, and they took my friend first. I lay in the ambulance thinking, "Hurry, hurry!" They took me second into the hospital. As they rolled my gurney along the corridor into surgery, I could only see the fluorescent lights passing on the ceiling. Still struggling to breathe, the surgeon appeared over my eyes, and I said to him, "You have permission to operate on me. This is my parent's phone number. Go to it!"

I awoke from surgery with my cousin Jeffrey holding my hand. He lived in San Francisco and was the first to come to my side. Later, my parents arrived, and I felt my mother squeeze my hand. She and I then knew I was going to survive.

The doctor told me the motorcycle's handlebar had broken my rib and ruptured my spleen. I was bleeding internally under my diaphragm, which explained why I experienced so much difficulty breathing. I received 14 blood transfusions, had my spleen removed, and lacerated my liver. My friend also underwent surgery, and fortunately, she lived to continue her life.

I share this event with you as it is a core motivating factor shaping my outlook. I have come to see life as a most precious, valuable gift. As in health, you only know what you've got once it's gone.

This event continues to shape and steer my life through happy coincidences, called synchronicities, leading me towards aiding others in any way I can and, ultimately in, raising your body's energy awareness. After the accident, I encountered an Acupressure Self-Massage book called "Do-In," compelling me to adopt a daily morning practice. Over five decades, I've added several key Yoga positions with Shiatsu and Isometrics into a 20-minute self-reliant routine, activating the body's energy meridians, enhancing and balancing vitality, and fostering a profound connection between physical, mental, and spiritual energy within our environment.

The Dynamic Self-Love Routine (DSLR) enhances health, vigor, and longevity and provides a daily practice to release the body from pain. Regularly practicing this routine energizes and harmonizes your bodily and spiritual being, removing energy blockages before they become chronic and ultimately attracting synchronicities for a richer and happier life. Pairing this energizing routine with a healthy diet and opening your awareness to the energies of our environment can profoundly enhance your life, fostering greater appreciation, joy, and success in living this life.

-INTRODUCTION-

DO-IN is an Ancient Chinese exercise routine focused on stimulating and balancing the energies within the human body. It was the source spring that aided in the discovery and application of Acupuncture so popular in the East and the West today.

DO-IN was first brought to the West by Frenchman Jacques de Langre in his book, *The First Book of DO-IN - Guide Pratique 1*, printed in 1971. I discovered this book in the 1970s. The book is both in French and English, teaching the various energetic movements and activities of DO-IN. For over 50 years I continually apply this daily practice.

His book, an 8" x 10" picture and illustration magazine, explains in great detail (inclusive of every energy meridian pathway) how energy flows through the body. *The Second Book of DO-IN* was published in 1974.

In the *Second Book of DO-IN*, the author suggested that the practice would also produce regeneration, health, and longevity. Following *The Second Book of DO-IN*, many other authors built upon the writings and practices of DO-IN, which are all available on Amazon.

Michio Kushi, in his book, *The Book of DO-IN: Exercise for Physical and Spiritual Development*, suggests that the practice would also enhance contact with the spiritual nature of man.

So the following offering is genuinely based upon the countless shoulders of other "Thinking Minds," who, through the ages, crafted imaginative thought and observation toward understanding the inner workings and nature of the human body.

While living in London as a psychologist working in three hospitals performing research for the National Health Service hospital system, I experienced constant annoying lower back pain. Dr. Alan Worsely, the founding discoverer who brought Acupuncture to the West, had a clinic in Coventry, a quaint English town north of London.

I went to Kings Cross station and bought a round-trip ticket, a yellow strip of thick, soft parchment-like paper, that gave me license to ride the smooth zoomy ride up to Coventry. His workman's era home was part of one long, red brick building, stretching along a whole city block. The building was a long construction of homes, doorway after doorway, with a dozen or more doors going along the entire length of a city block. This area had blocks and blocks of the same construction of buildings. Stepping into his modest home, he led me to the first room on the left, a small heated room containing a leather massage table covered with a thick, soft, white cover.

In one corner on the left sat a small, brown, circular wooden table supporting a lamp covered by a light reddish cloth. The cloth on the light gave off a diminished golden-reddish hue bathing the room. What immediately hit my senses was that the room smelled of a very subtle sweet jasmine scent.

Bang! I was in!

He asked me why I had come to him. I told him I had pain in my lower back. He asked me if he could hold my hand. I gave him my left hand, and he held it in his left hand. With his right hand, he took his second, third, and fourth fingers and placed them on specific points on my wrist.

He then had me lie on the table and placed several needles gently into my back. He then instructed me to relax for about 15 minutes. He then returned, removed the needles, and explained that he had completed my treatment.

I asked if I needed to return, and he said, "No."

I asked, "That's it?"

He replied, "Yes, you're done, and you won't need further treatments."

He asked me to pay £15 British Pounds for his services. After which I returned to London. While walking to my flat, I felt a sudden surge of energy shooting directly into the pain in my back, and it was gone! This back pain didn't return for many, many years.

I offer this story to help you understand my motivations in sharing the following ancient, inner-directed, self-healing knowledge with you.

Why do the Following Exercises?

Acupressure, which is acupuncture without using needles, offers you the power to create health and vigor in your body. This routine will balance and invigorate all the internal energy pathways. These internal energy pathways are called meridians of energy flow in acupuncture. These exercises will stimulate the meridians which reinvigorate the body energy pathways to promote well-being and health. Through years of extensive research, acupuncture has become a firmly established medical alternative to many modern Western Medicines.

Pay attention to any painful areas in your body during this process. Pain indicates that your energy flow in these areas are blocked. Take extra time to stimulate these areas through deeper, circular massage (explained further in the following section). Eventually, you will be able to mitigate these painful areas and increase joyful flexibility and vitality.

I'm confident committing yourself every morning to these energizing exercises will hook you into how enjoyable it is being connected to your body. Eventually unexpected nourishing events will start entering your life. (further discussed in Chapter 3). Synchronicity is significant occurrences of events that enter and nourish your life without any conscious effort. This term was coined by Dr. Carl Jung in Switzerland through his study of symbols in the 1950's.

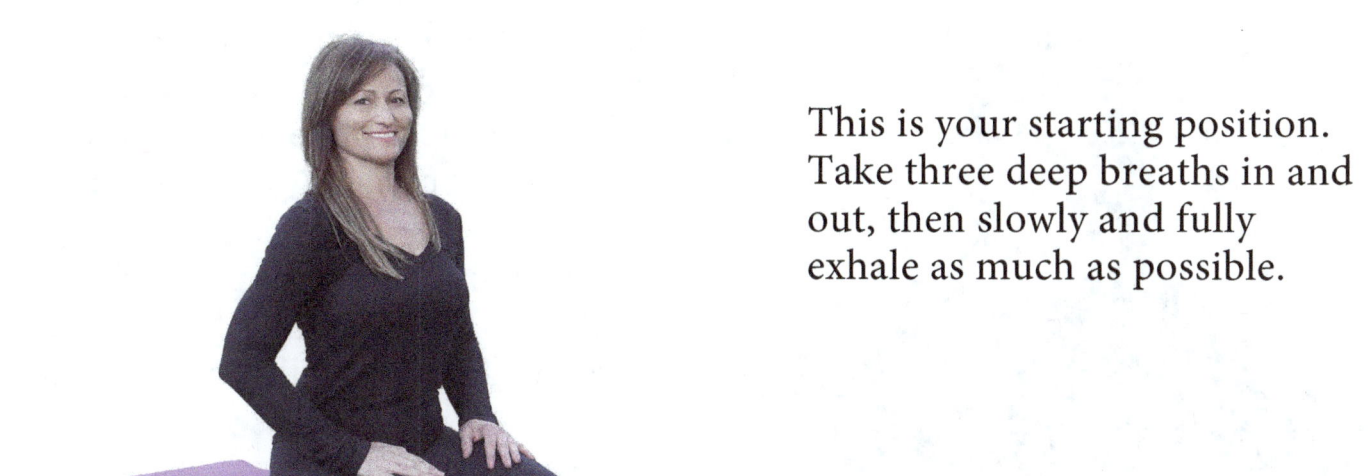

This is your starting position. Take three deep breaths in and out, then slowly and fully exhale as much as possible.

As you exhale, bow forward, touching the tips of your thumb and index finger together, making a triangle shape while placing your forehead between your hands.

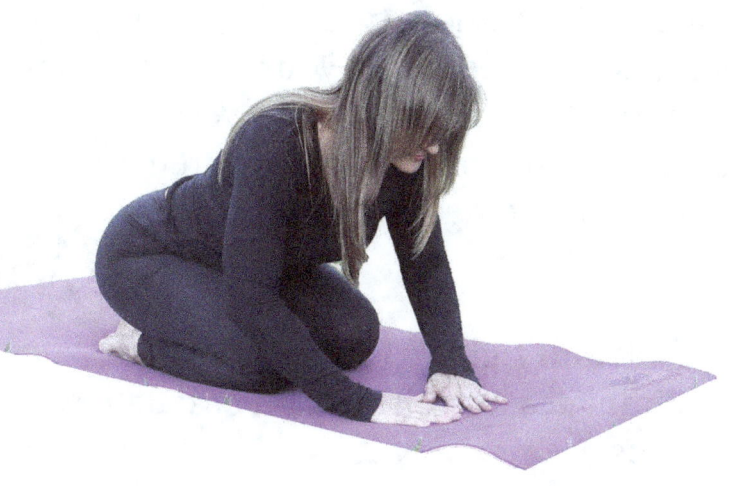

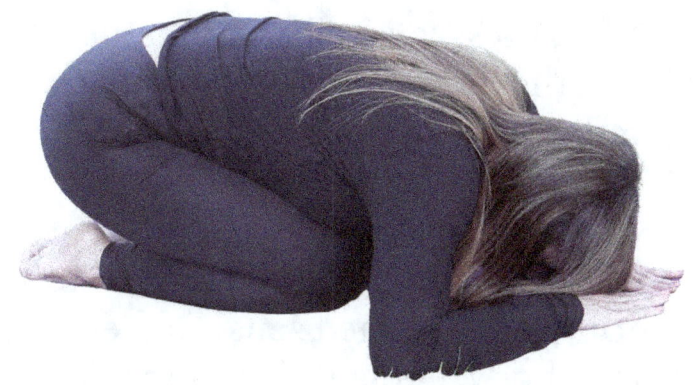

Exhale fully, placing your forehead into the triangle in front of you. Exhale as deeply as possible and hold as long as you can as this will empty your lungs and make them ready to oxygenate your body and wake you up.

Then rise, taking a deep breath inward, filling your lungs and chest as fully as possible.

4

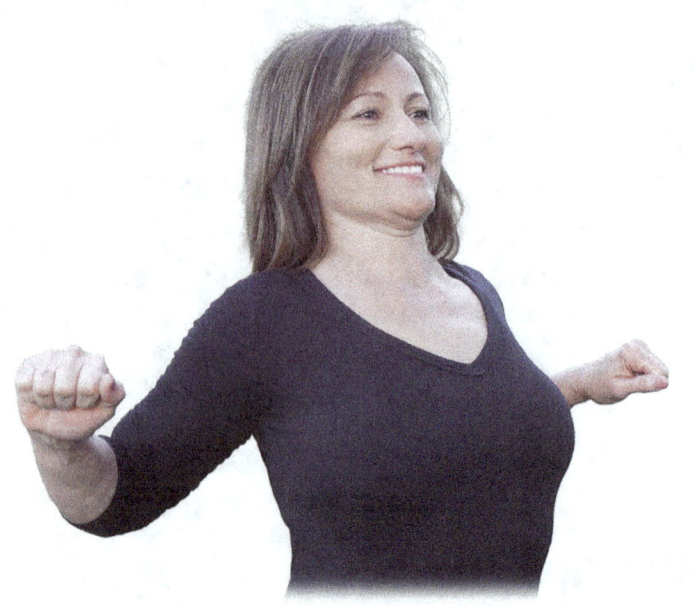

On this stretch, bring your elbows and shoulders as close together behind you. Feel this stretch move down from your neck and shoulders, into your spine.

Stretch your chest outward while inhaling. This stimulates the bladder meridian and lubricates the spinal disks.

While in this position, twist left and right. Feel this stretch deeply in your back muscles throughout the entire length of your spine. This movement enhances the awareness of feeling the strength of your spine.

Swing left and right to the count of 20. This stimulates lung, heart and circulatory meridians.

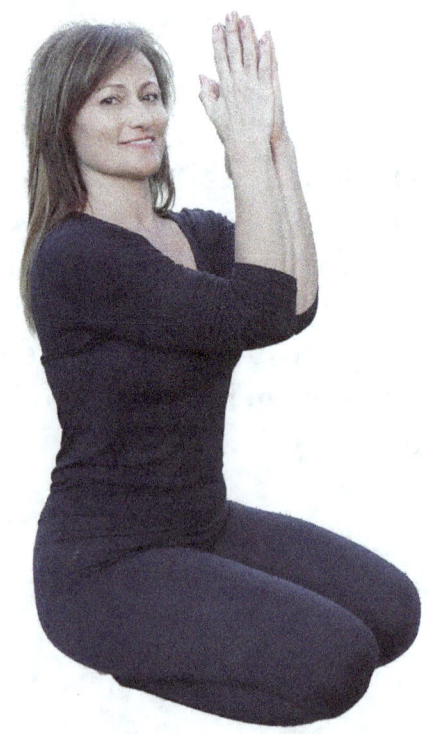

Next, press your elbows together. Feel the tension in your shoulders and neck. Do this stretch to the count of 20.

All these stretches are designed to bring a heightened sense of feeling to your body, and stimulates the respiratory, intestinal, heart and circulatory systems.

5

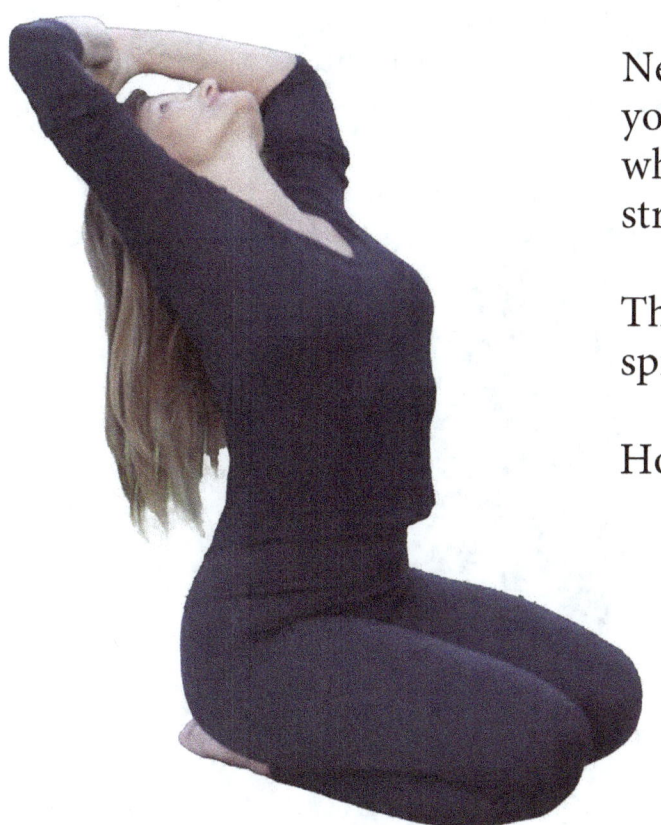

Next, interlace your fingers together above your head. Stretch as far back as possible, while tilting your head back-wards. Feel the stretch in your neck and down your spine.

This stretch travels all the way down the spine.

Hold to the count of 20.

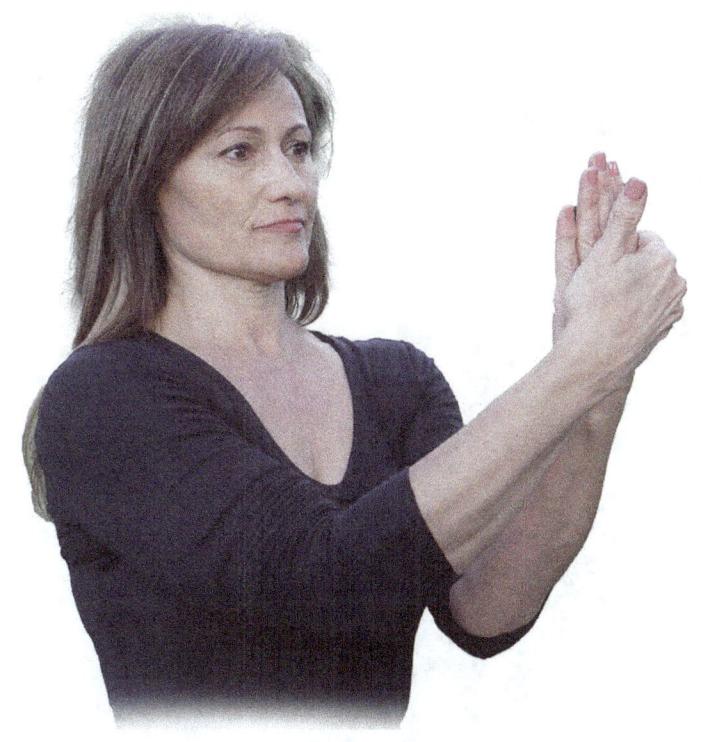

Grab the front of your left hand and twist it inward while pulling your hand into the chest five times.

You should feel the stretch moving deeply toward the shoulder blade and back. This stimulates also the cardiac, respiratory, digestive, and circulatory meridians.

While twisting your hand outward, bring your pinkie towards your chest. Feel the stretch travel up the arm and into your shoulder blade. This movement stretches your arm into the back of your shoulder, and stimulates heart and lung meridians. Perform the same movement with your right arm.

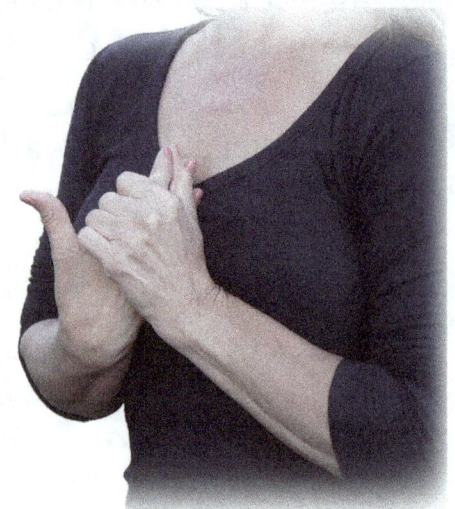 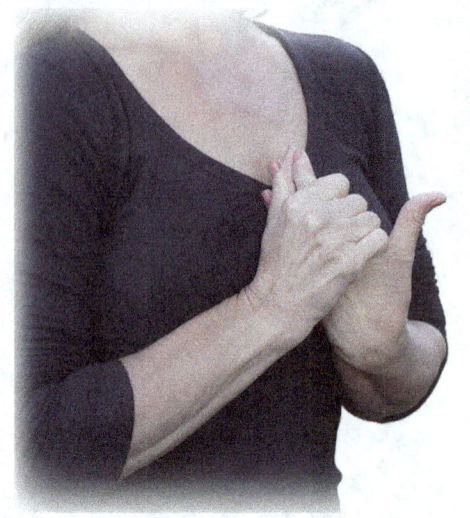

Next, clap your hands together and rub them briskly and vigorously. This energizes the tools you are going to use to heal your body. You are going to seek out tender or painful areas, to massage them and free energy blockages.

Clap, rub, and shake your hands often through out the exercises to energize the healing power of your hands.

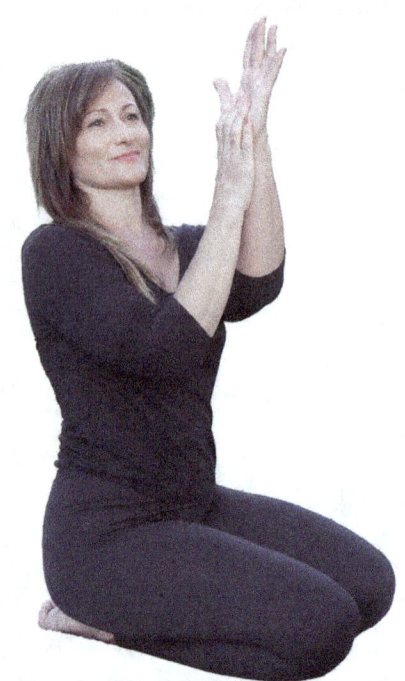

Next, shake your hands back and forth, freely from the wrists to raise energy and power within your hands, arms, shoulders and back.

You will begin to feel the flow of energy increasing from this stimulation.

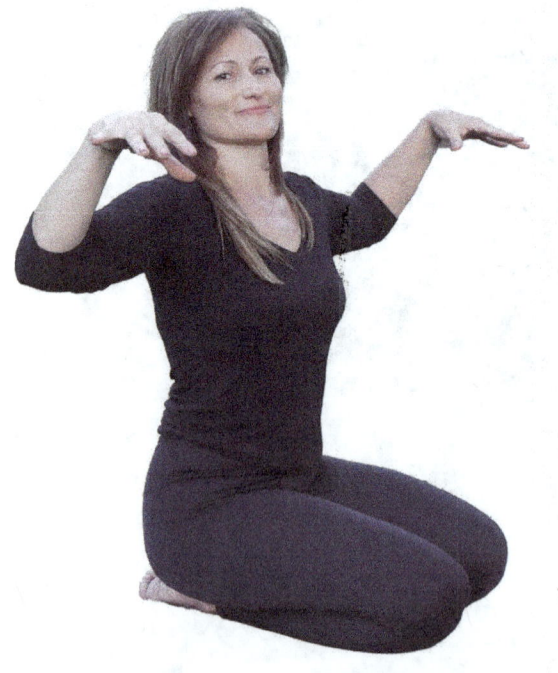

7

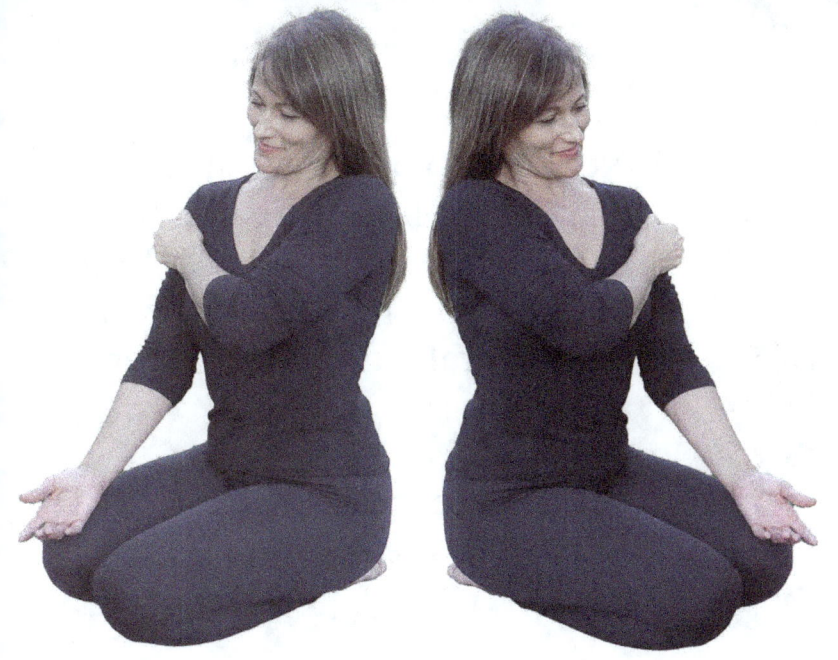

Use your hand to form a fist and pound behind your shoulder moving down, pounding the whole length of your arm, towards your fingertips. This invigorates the respiratory, circulatory, cardiac, and digestive meridians.

Repeat the same action on both arms as shown

Next, jam your fingers together repeatedly, interlacing them as shown. Draw your fingers apart and then jam them back together repeatedly 20 times.

This stimulates energy all the way up your arms and into your shoulders and back.

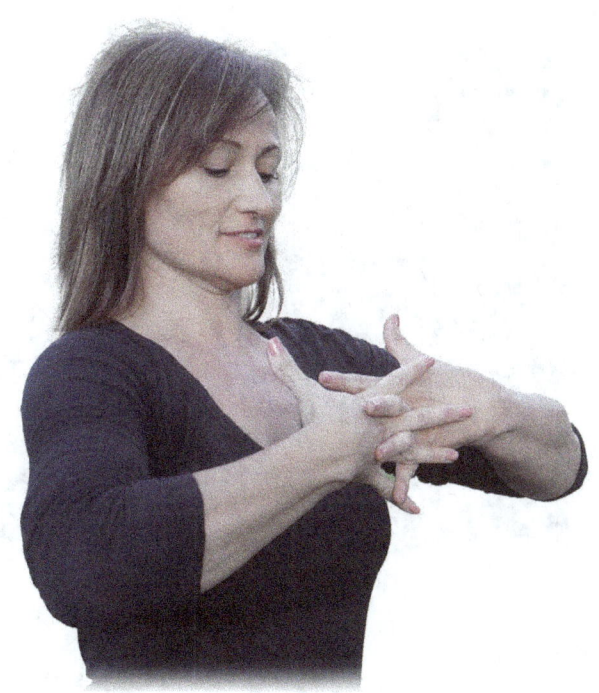

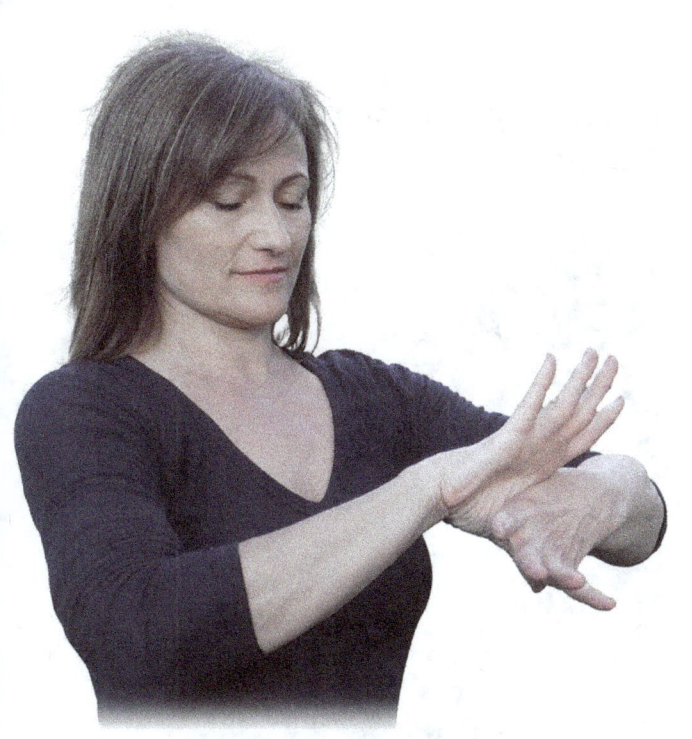

Then, jam the the space between your thumb and index fingers together, repeatedly for 20 times.

This energizes your hands and arms simultaneously.

8

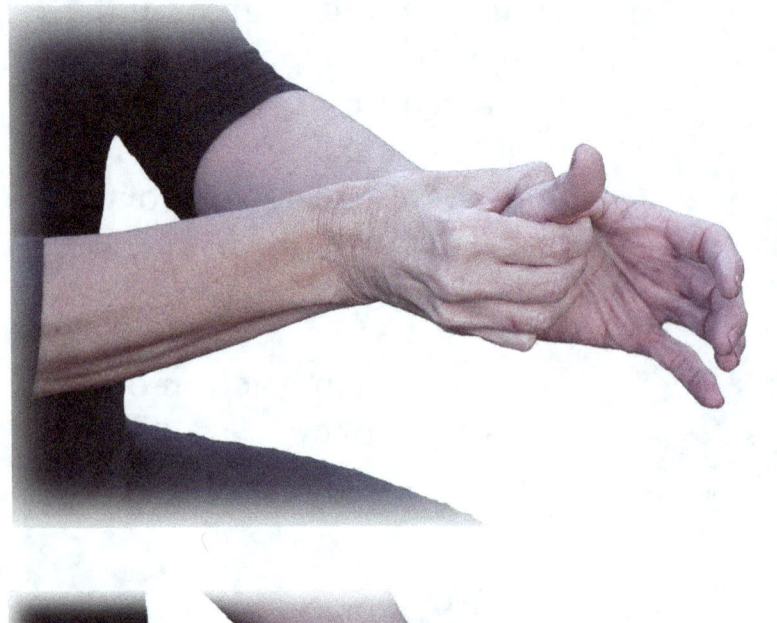

Next, take your four fingers and place them into the palm of your hand, while pressing your thumb on the opposite side, between your thumb and index finger as shown.

Massage in a clockwise circular motion to the count of 20.

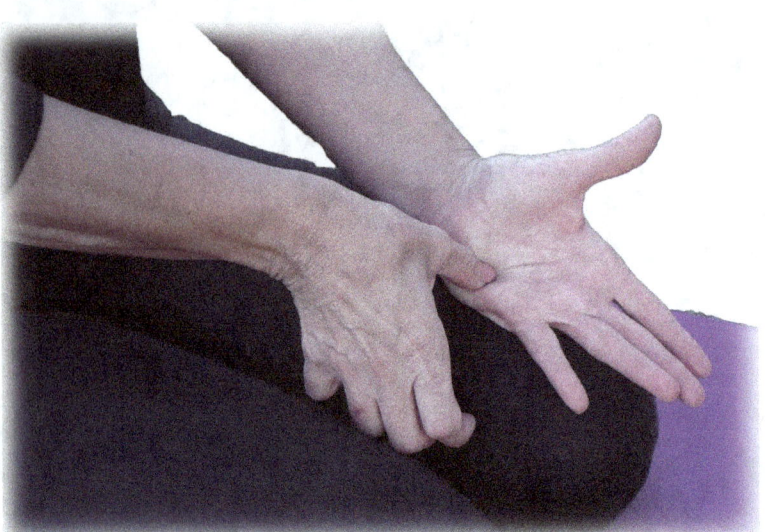

Next, use your thumb to massage this portion of your hand, as shown. This sends energy through your heart meridian, the acupressure energy flow leading to your heart.

Massage in a clockwise circular motion, counting to 20. Repeat the entire massage on the opposite hand.

Now, gently pinch each individual fingertip while making circular movements to each finger.

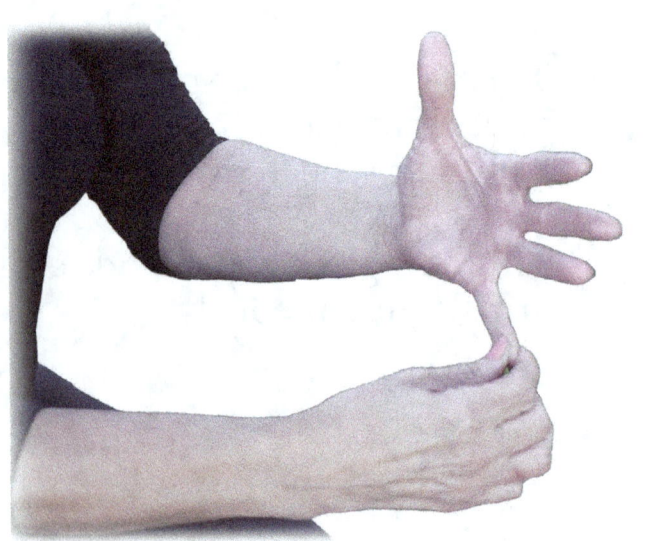
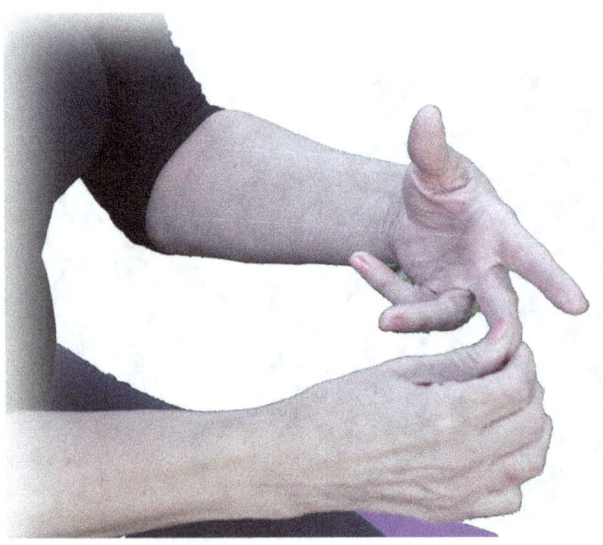

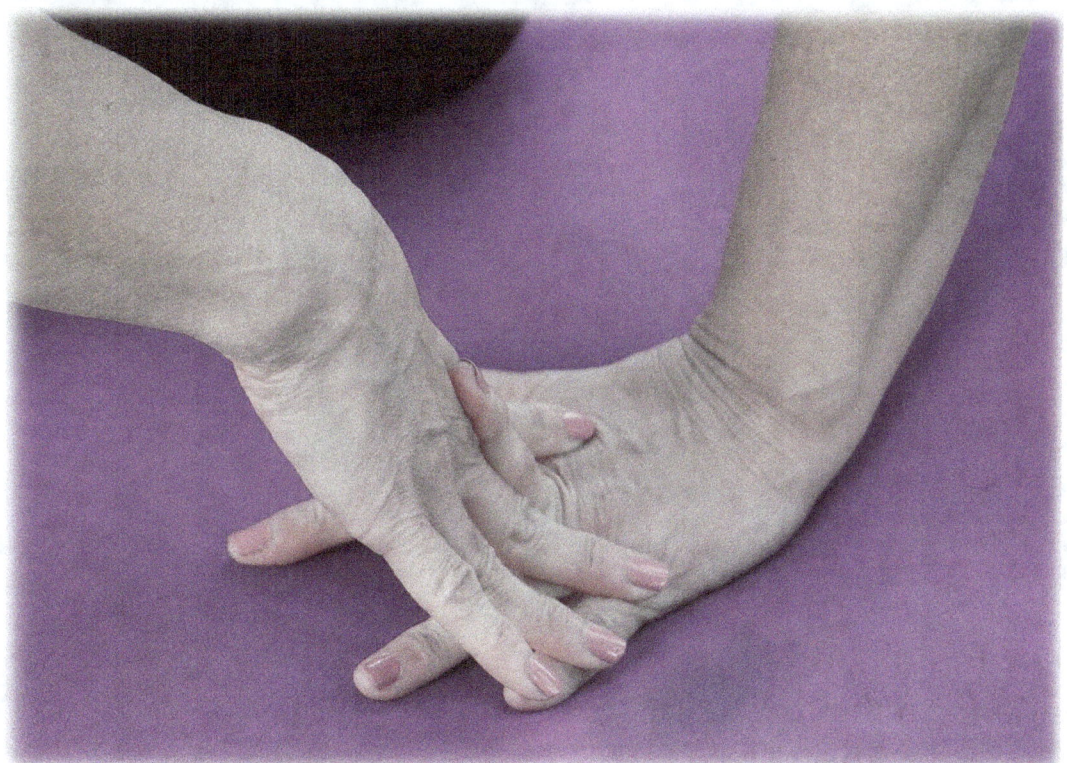

Next, place your left hand sideways on the floor with your fingers and thumb spread out. Use your right hand, interlaced, to lift one individual finger upward at a time. Allow each finger and thumb to snap back down to the floor. This will test whether any pains exist, indicating a lack of balance in the cardiac, respiratory, digestive and circulatory meridians. Repeat on the other hand.

Allow each finger to snap back to the floor, sending energy all the way up the arm.

Next, pinch each fingertip twice across the nail. In a single motion, pinch and pull each fingertip outward, letting each pinch slip out in a snapping motion. This sends energy from your fingertips into the rest of your body

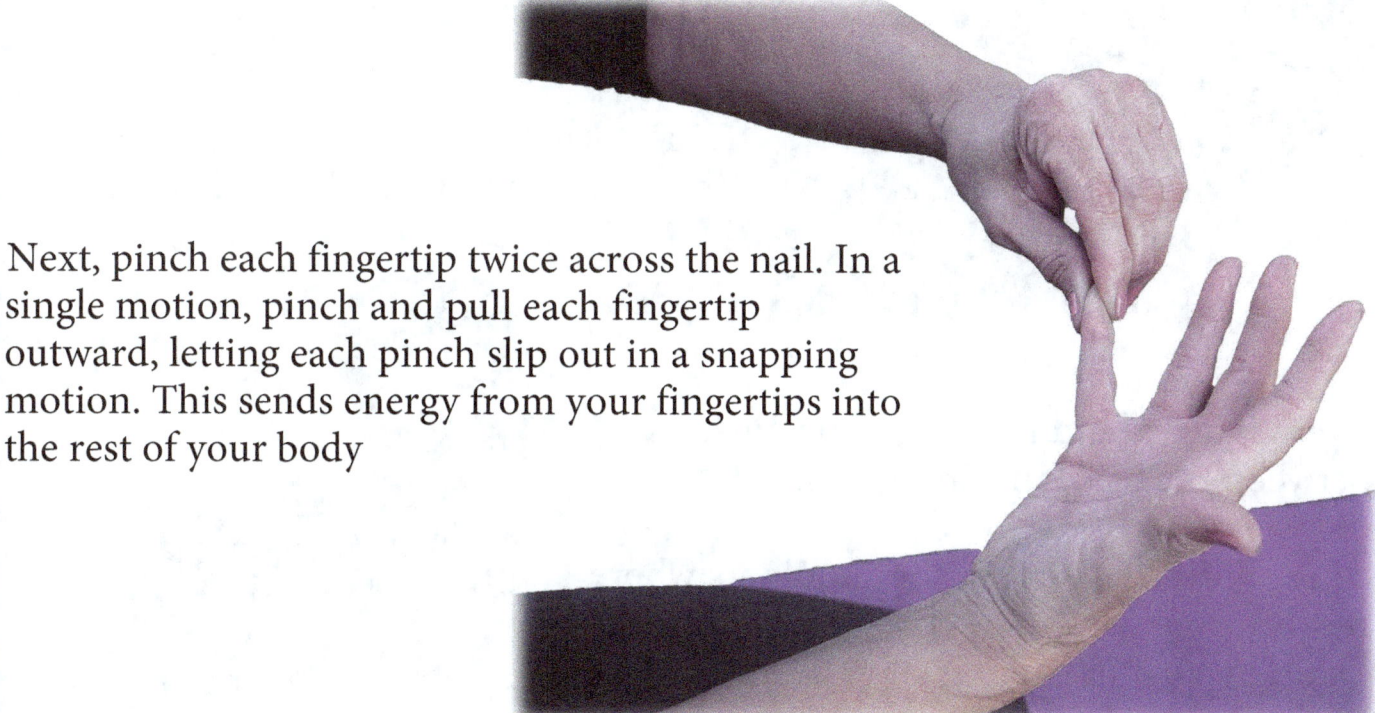

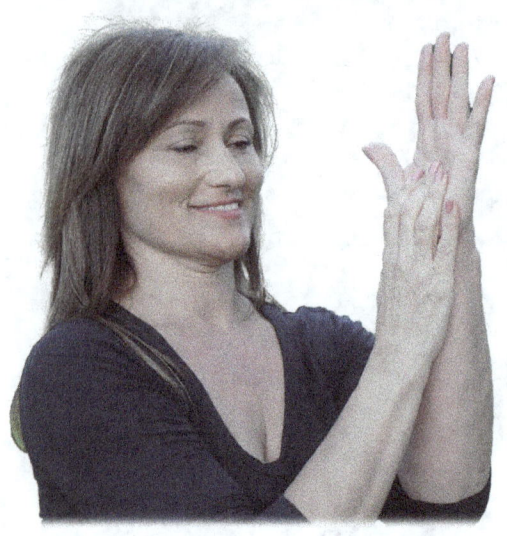

Now, rub, slap, and shake your hands together again to revitalize the energy in your hands.

Do this to the count of 20.

Next, with your thumbs, find two small indentations on the back of your skull. Place your fingertips along the top of your head.
With all your fingers, massage these areas in a circular motion to the count of 20.
This stimulates many meridians in your body.

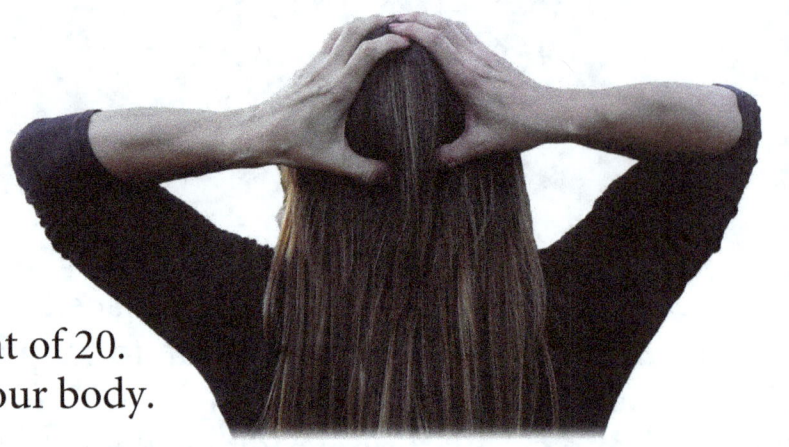

Next, while tilting your head forward, find an opening between the back of your skull and your neck. Massage this area in a circular motion. This stimulates the brain stem. Follow by massaging the entire neck.

This releases tension and stimulates the flow of energy in the neck area.

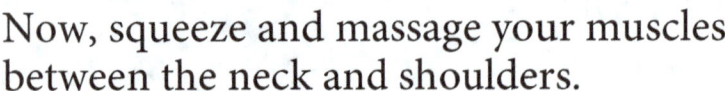

Now, squeeze and massage your muscles between the neck and shoulders.

This releases tension in the shoulders where most people feel strain. This increases flexibility and awareness of your back.

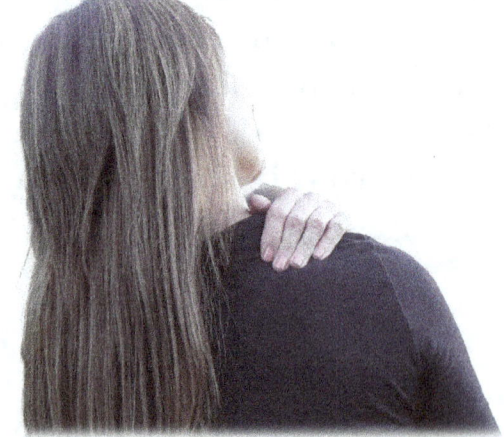

11

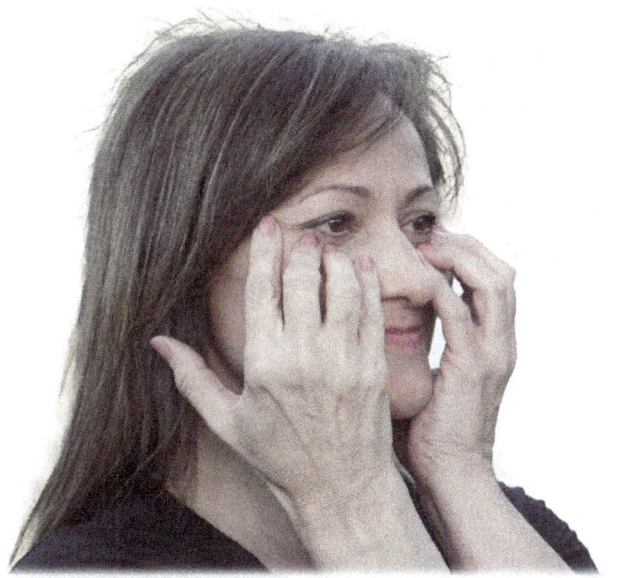

Next, use your fingertips to stimulate your entire face. Draw your fingertips downward, from your forehead to your chin, repeating multiple times. Then, in a circular motion, massage above your eyebrows and below your eyes. Squeeze the bridge of the nose. This delivers energy from your hands to your face.

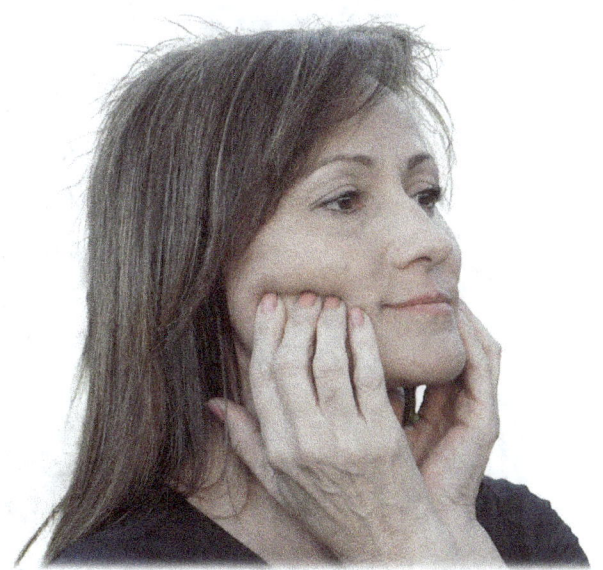

Now, massage the upper and lower jaw and gums using your fingertips in a circular motion. This massage increases blood flow into your gums and teeth, while promoting digestive health.

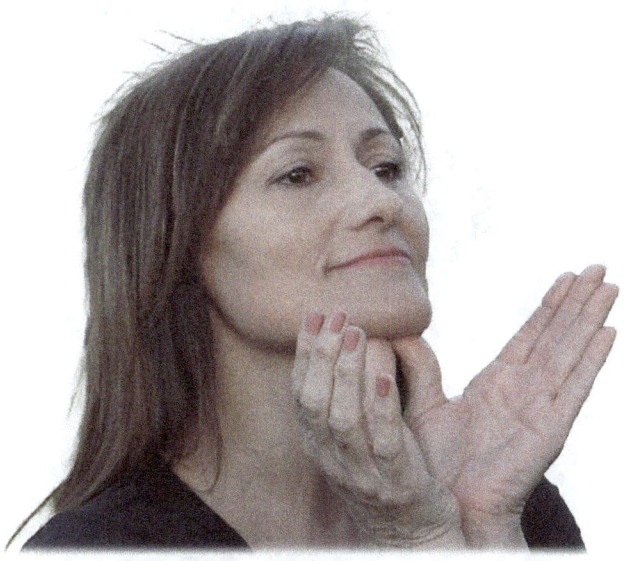

Next, use your thumbs in a circular motion to massage the soft tissue underneath the chin. This mitigates over-eating and helps prevent a double chin.

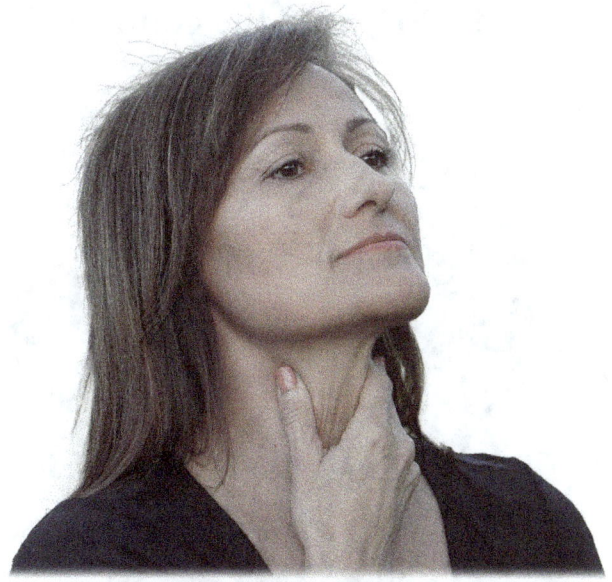

Then gently stimulate the thyroid gland by squeezing and rubbing both sides of the throat area.

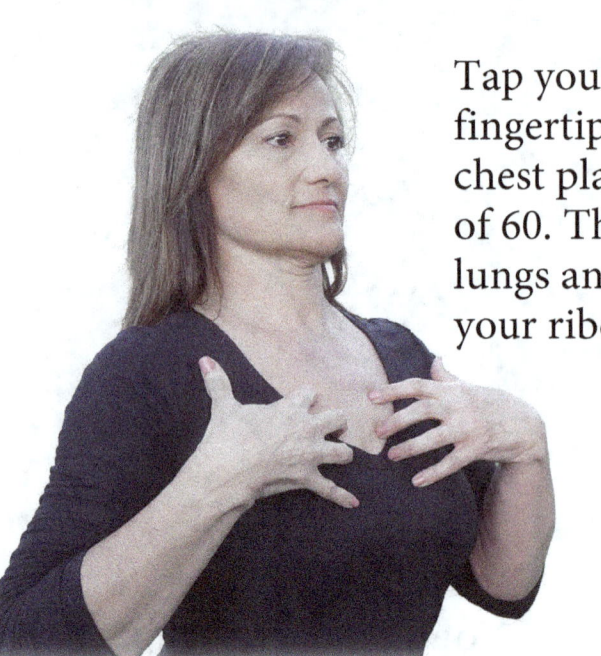

Tap your chest with your fingertips all over your chest plate for the count of 60. This stimulates the lungs and awareness of your ribcage area.

Next, in circular motion, use your fingertips to massage your abdomen. Move left and right and go as deep as you comfortably can to massage, activate, and stimulate your internal organs. Do this to the count of 20. Seek any painful areas and give them additional attention.

Next, use your fingertips or closed hands to gently tap around your head. Do this to the count of 20. This stimulates the cranial meridians.

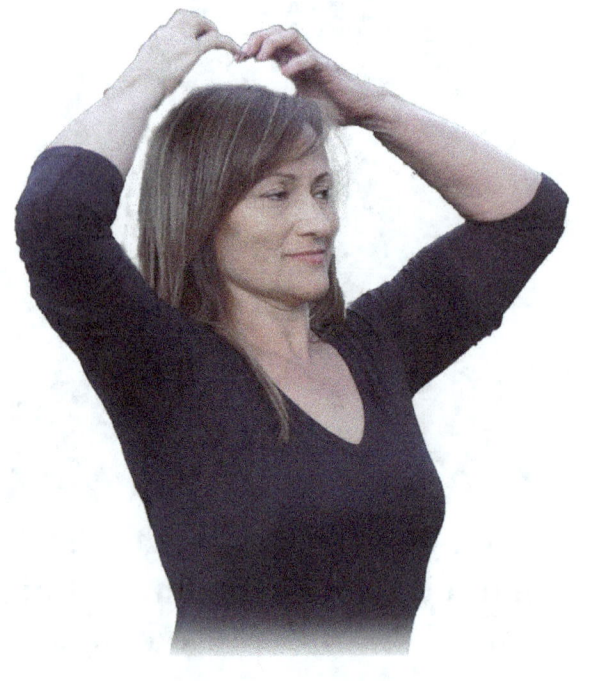

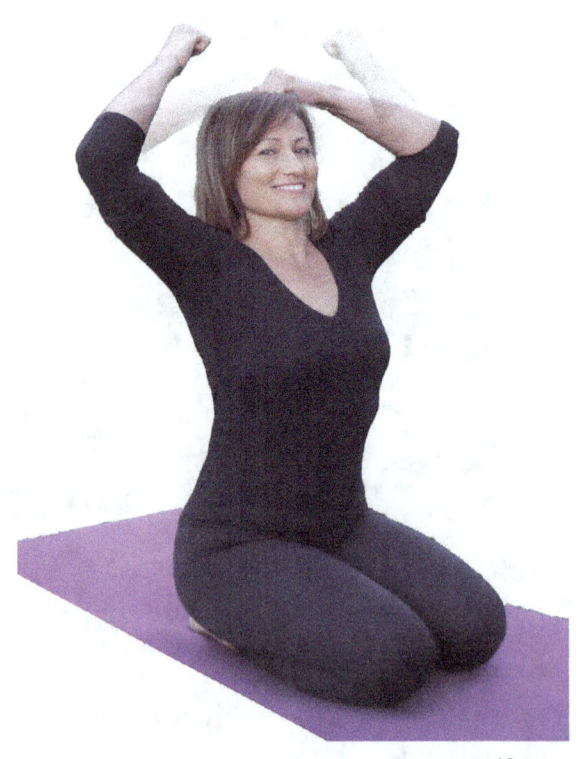

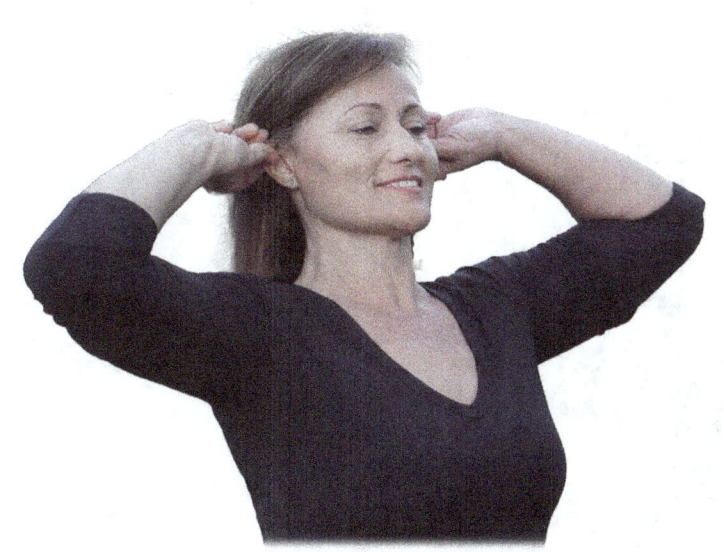

Next, massage your ears.
Pull your ears up and down, running your fingers inside and outside.

You will immediately feel a strong sense of energy being released from this massage, due to the numerous meridians in the earlobes.

After massaging your ears, cross your ankles and grab your feet. Start rolling along your back until you reach your shoulders.

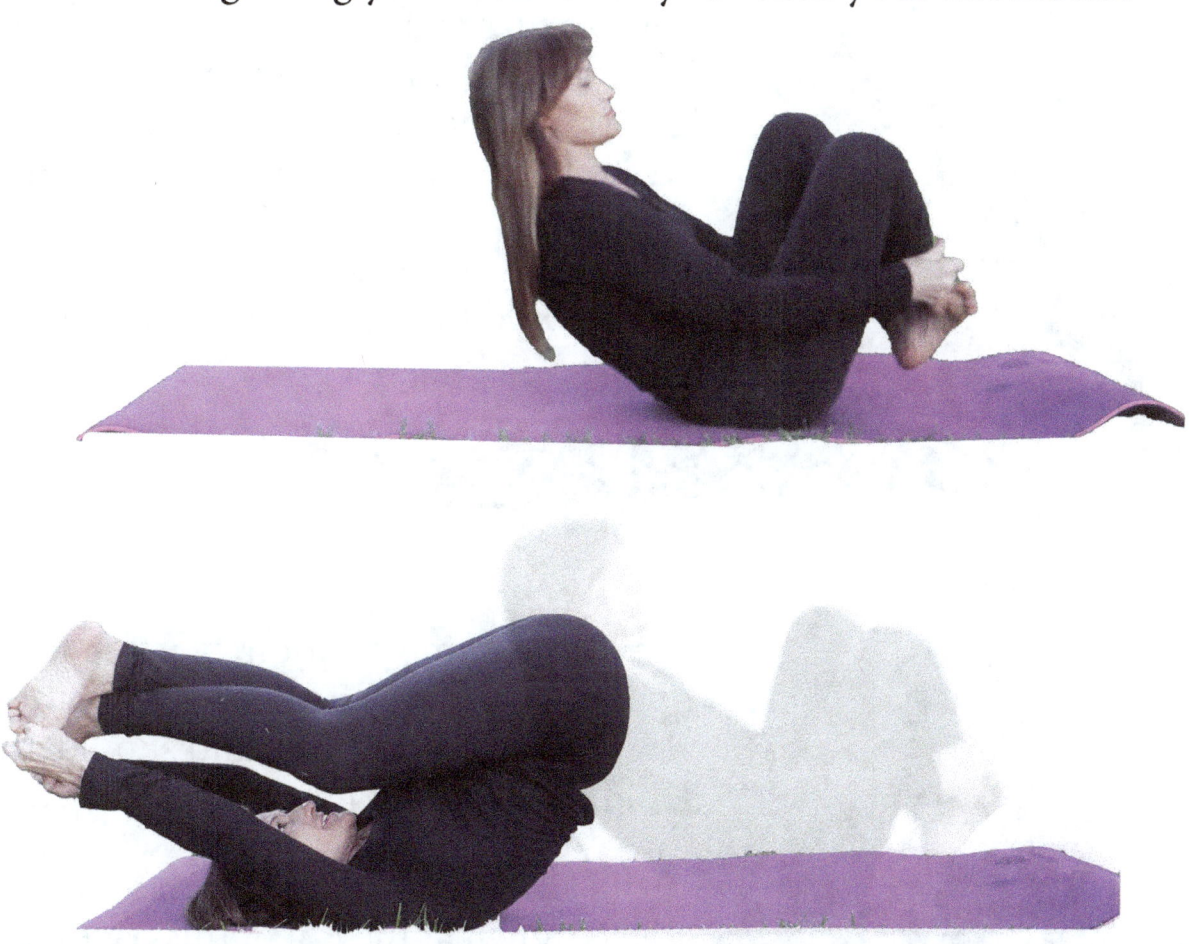

Once you rolled upon your shoulders, roll back to the starting position. Repeat this exercise by rolling back and forward. The goal is to massage and energize your entire back. This stimulates the brain and spinal chord nerve pathways. Rock back and forth for 20 repetitions.

Place your legs straight in front of you. Lean forward as far as you can to stretch your lower back. Count to 20 in this position. The goal is to stretch forward by pulling yourself to go as low as comfortable. This promotes flexibility, stretching the spinal disks and back muscles.

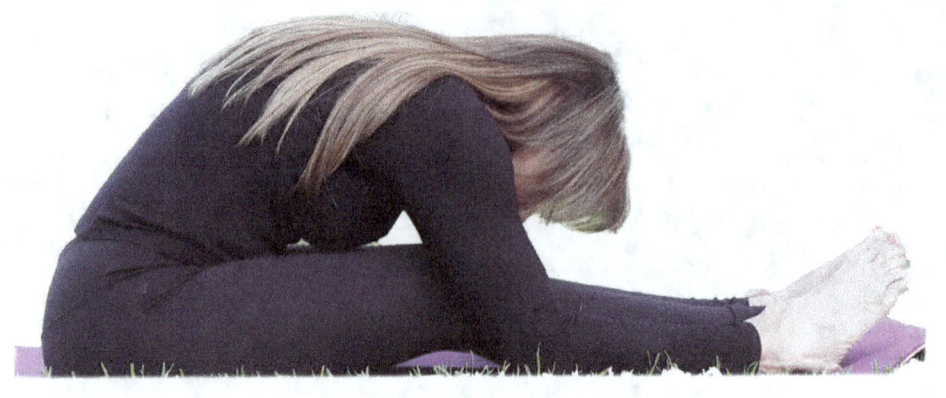

Next, twist your shoulders to look left behind you while placing your right leg over your left as show Use your right elbow as leverage to press against t right knee while looking backward. This is to twis and stretch your spine, neck and sholders.

Only go as far as you are comfortable. Hold this position to the count of 20.

Repeat the same position, twisting in the opposite direction. This stimulates the right side of your spine, neck, and shoulder muscles. Hold this position for the count of 20.

Once completed, return to the position shown at the top of this page, repeating the entire sequence 3 times, counting to 20 at each of the three stretches.

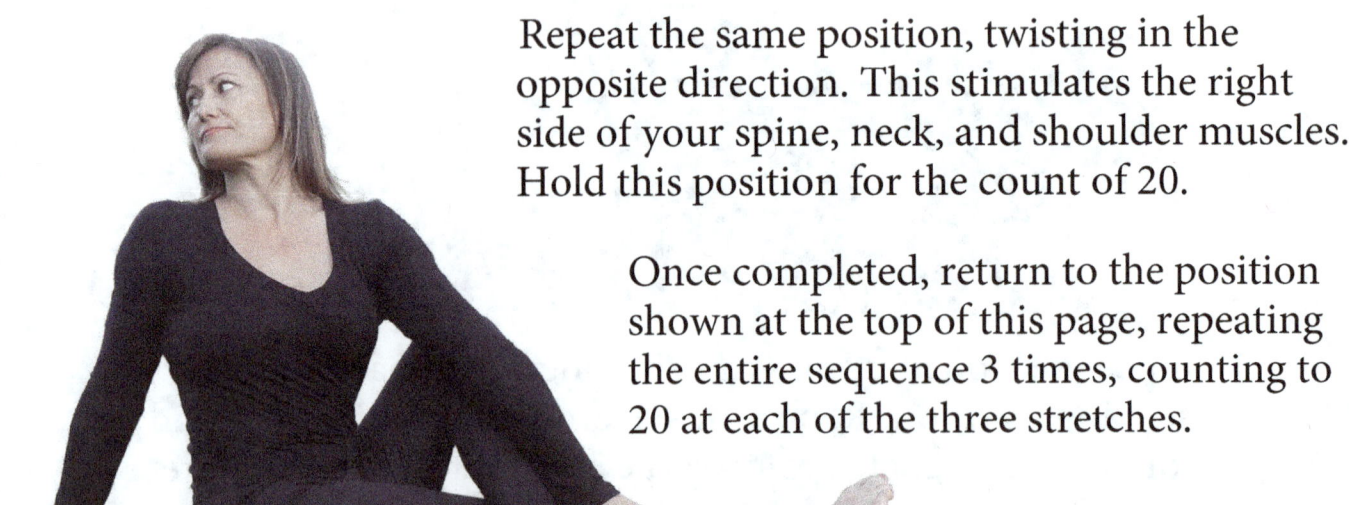

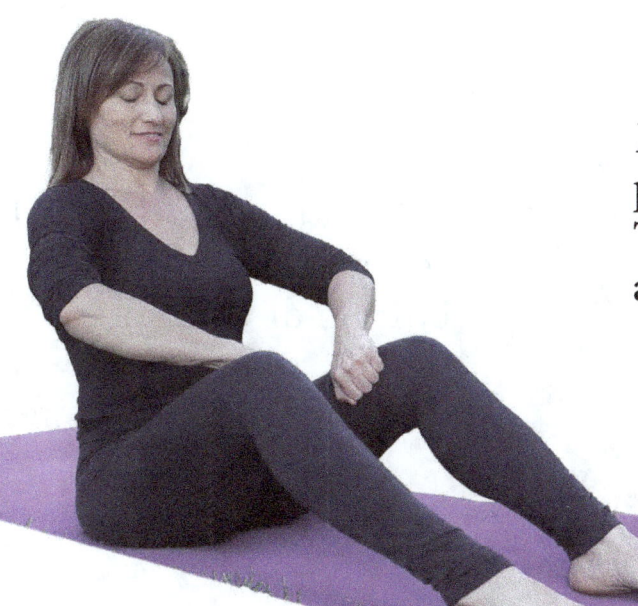

Make fists with your hands and start pounding the inside of your thighs. Travel downward to your calf muscles and then to your ankles.

Repeat this percussive massage on the outside of your thighs, traveling down through the outside of your calves and ankles.

This is to stimulate and increase blood flow and awareness of your legs. This promotes digestion and lessens fatigue by activating and balancing the meridians.

Next, rub and gently pinch the Achilles tendon, either by rubbing or squeezing the area shown to the right.

This releases a flow of energy into the foot and up the leg. Repeat this massage on both feet.

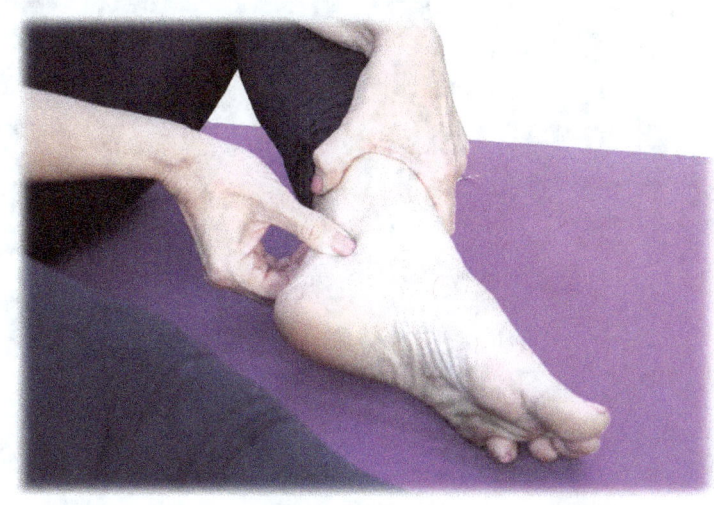

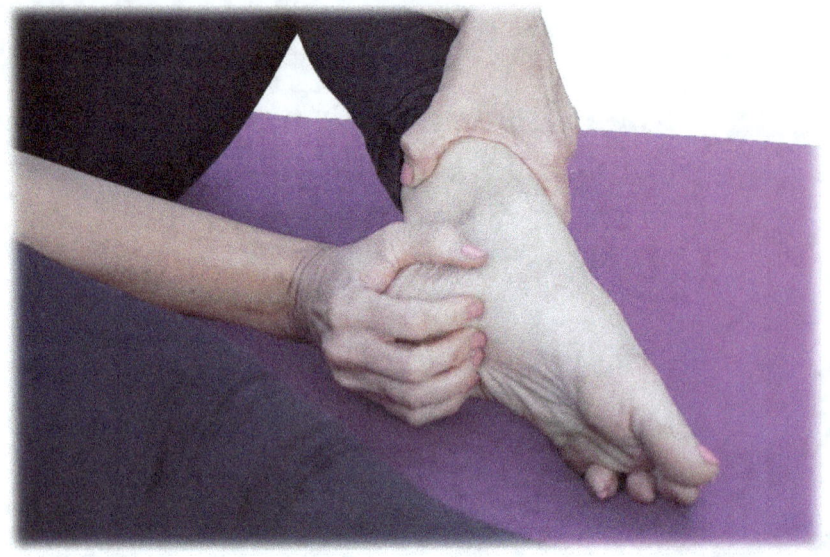

Next, squeeze your heel firmly several times to stimulate the bottom of your foot, as shown.

This stimulates bone formation.

Then make a fist. Use your knuckles to rub and massage the underside of your foot, as shown. Move up and down in circular motions.

The goal is to stimulate the bottom of the entire foot because all the acupressure meridians reside in the bottom of the foot. You can stimulate your entire body by just rubbing your feet.

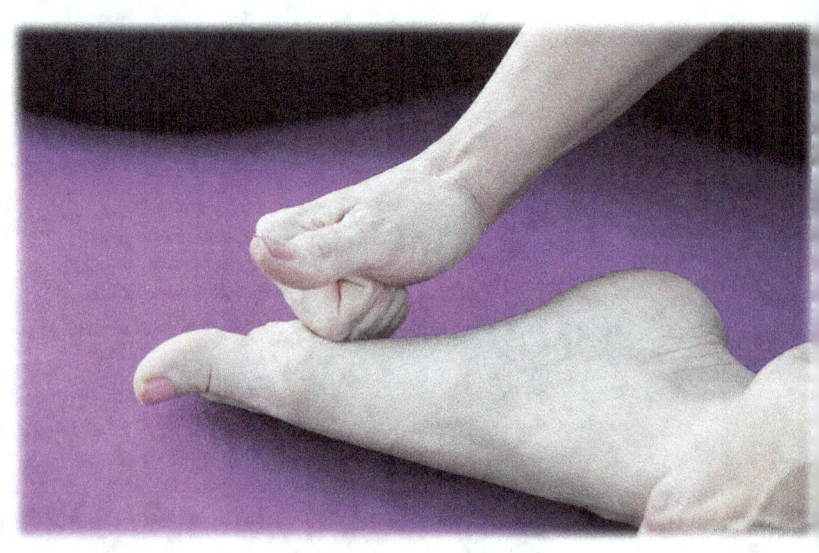

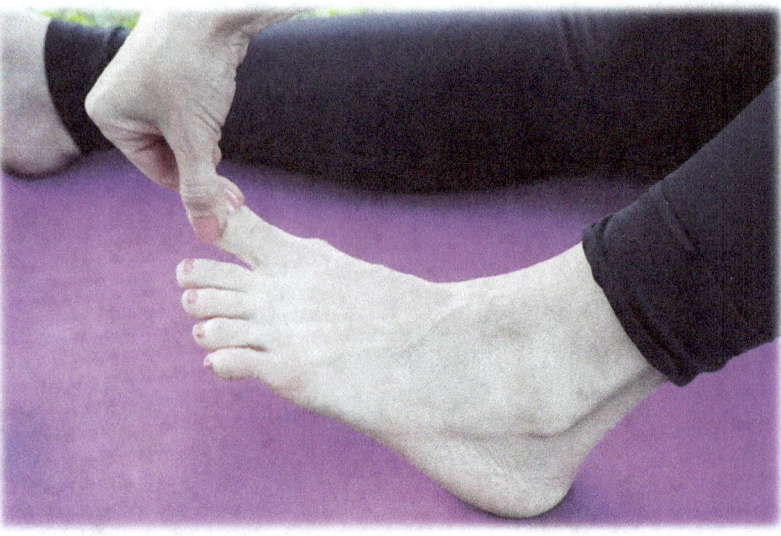

Repeat the same massage we did with your fingers, but with your toes. Use your index finger and thumb, to rub and wiggle each toe.

In a pulling motion, snap the end of each toe on either side of the nail, twice, causing energy to release from the toes.

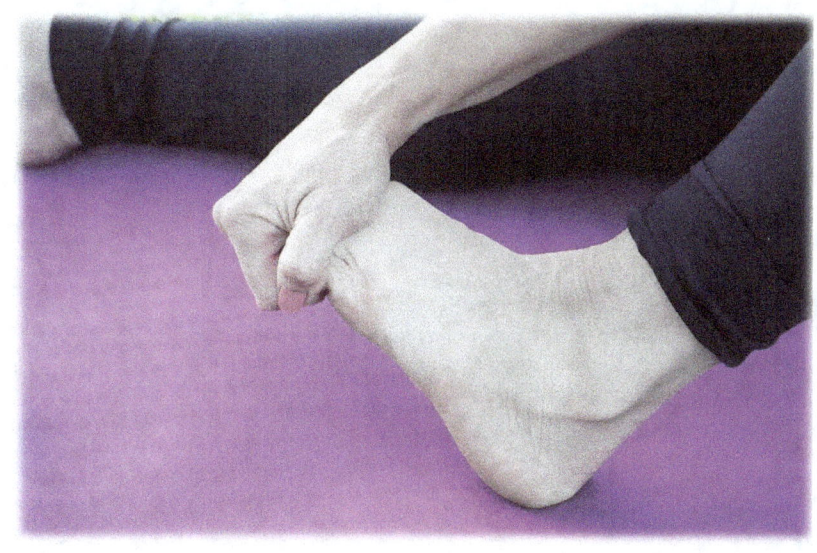

After pulling the toes, grab all 5 toes and curl them downward. Next, use your palm to slap the bottom of the foot 10 times to stimulate energy.

Afterward, toss your foot outward while extending the leg. Repeat the above on the other foot.

Next, sit on you knees to stretch your arms forwards as far as possible, as shown. Then rise forward on your hands and knees, moving back and forth 10 times. This stretches your arms, shoulders, back and hips in one fluid motion, and releases the flow of energy into your entire body.

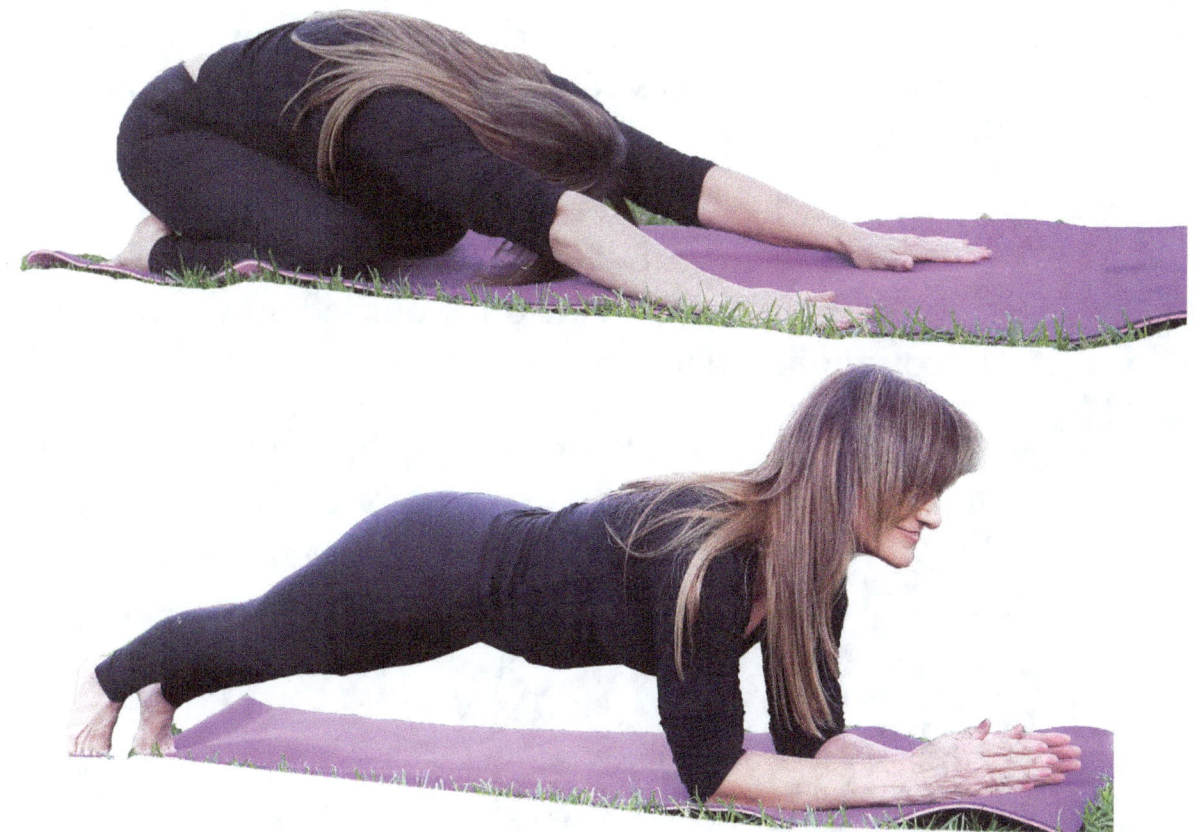

Next, do the plank. This strengthens the entire body from neck to toes, and all muscles in between. Hold this position with the goal of counting to 60. Holding this position fires all the muscle groups simultaneously, benefiting posture, balance, coordination, spine alignment, building core strength, flexibility, metabolism, and mental health.

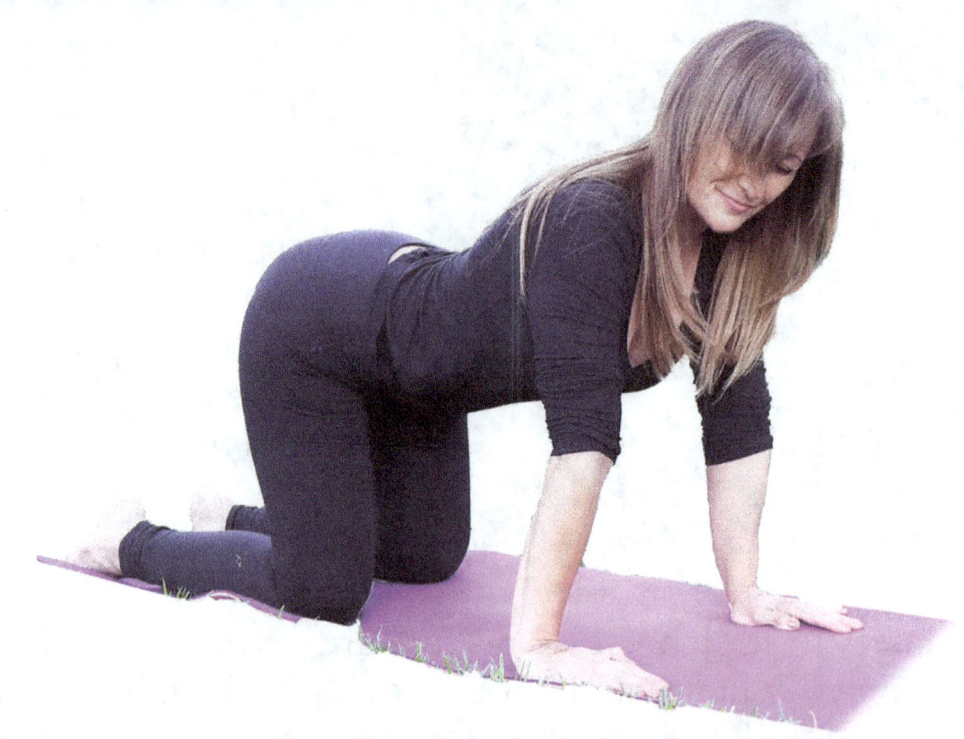

On your hands and knees, twist, bend and shake your spine and neck so you can release energy into your head, neck, shoulders, spine, and hips. Do this motion to experience your body as one single flow of motion. This releases tension and enhances contact with your body. Do this movement to the count of 20.

Next, stretch each leg by kicking upward and behind, in an alternating motion, kicking your left and right legs to the count of 20. This energizes the spine, hips, legs, arms, and ne

Note: Unlike the illustration, keep your elbows straight to allow energy to flow from shoulders to fingertips.

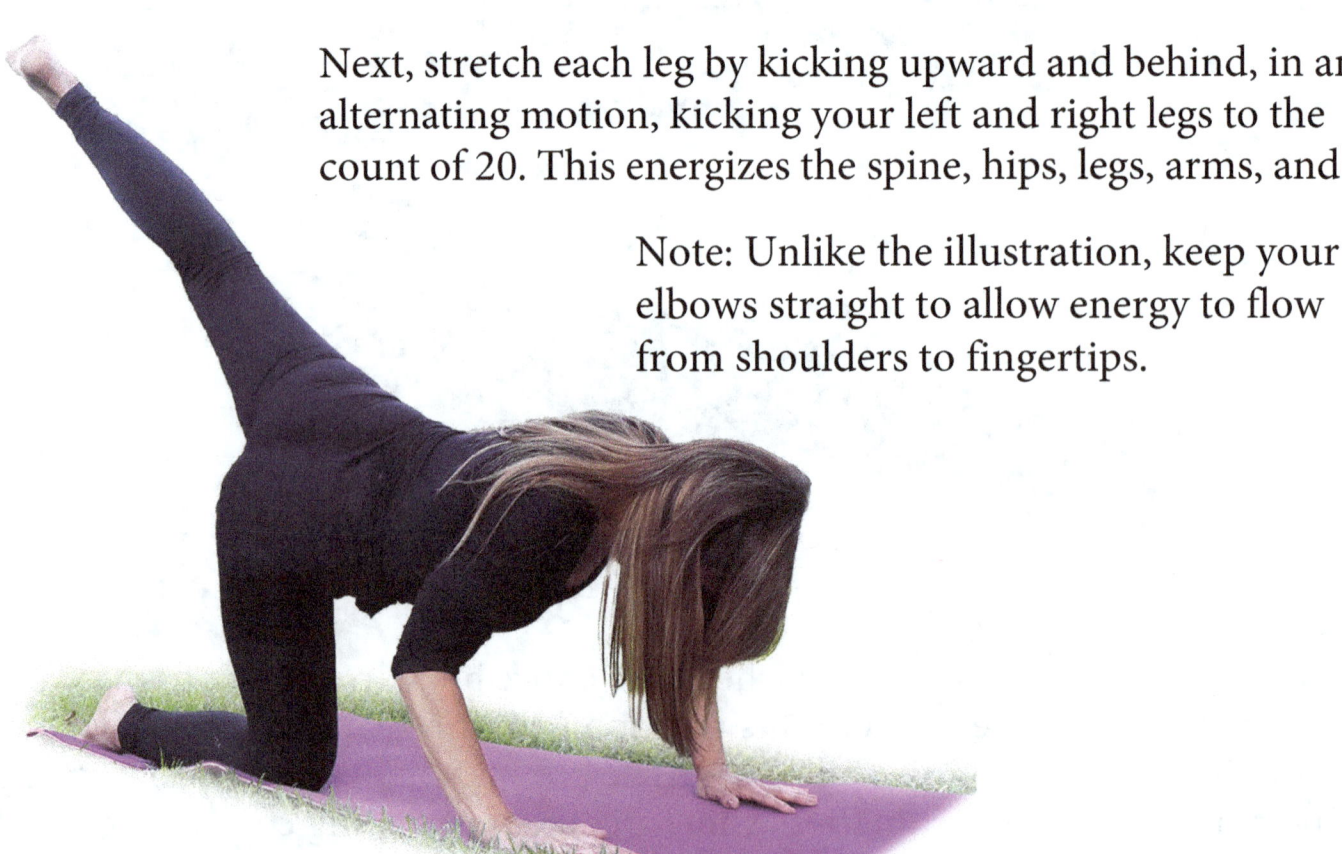

These are two separate exercises. While lying on your back, move your legs as if you are peddling a bicycle. Do this to the count 20. This stimulates your knees.

Next, stretch both legs outward, then move each leg up and down almost touching the floor and then back up, as pictured below. Do this to the count of 20. This stimulates the hips.

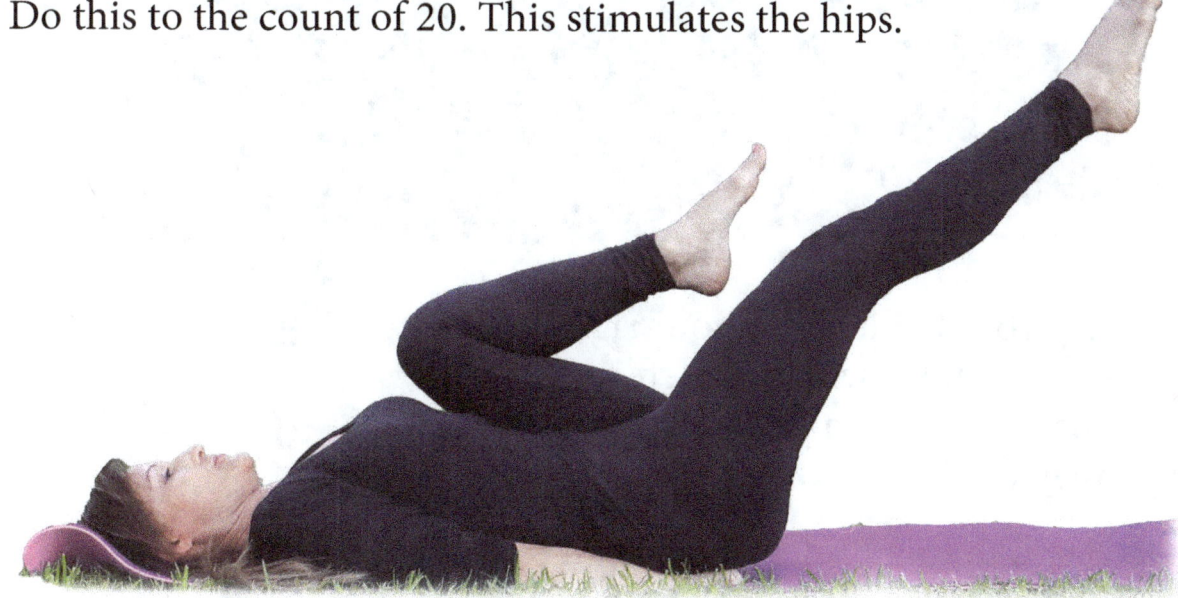

While on your back, holding your legs by the knees, roll your body left and right. This massage stimulates your back, shoulders, hips, and spine, and activates the spinal cord meridian running along your back.

Rock left and right to the count of 20.

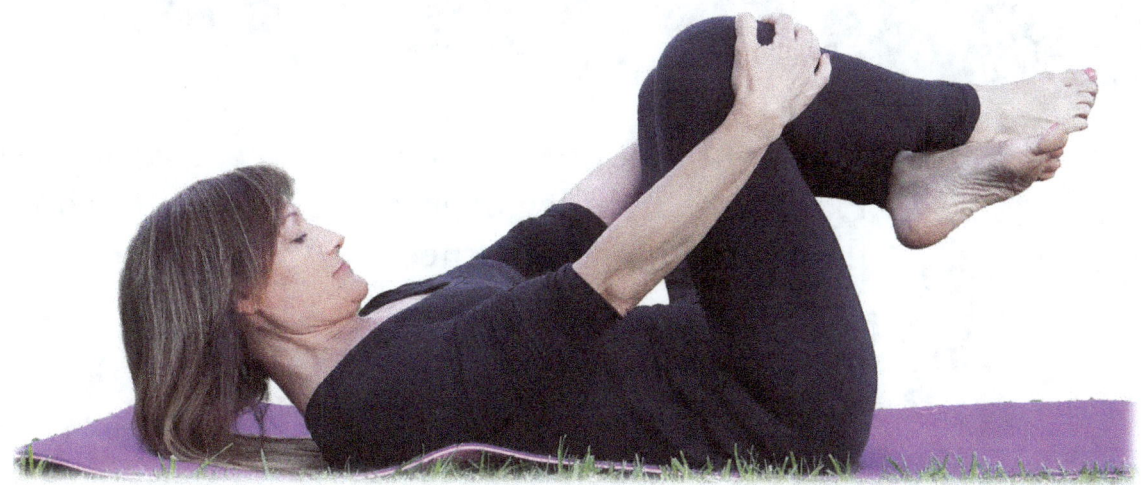

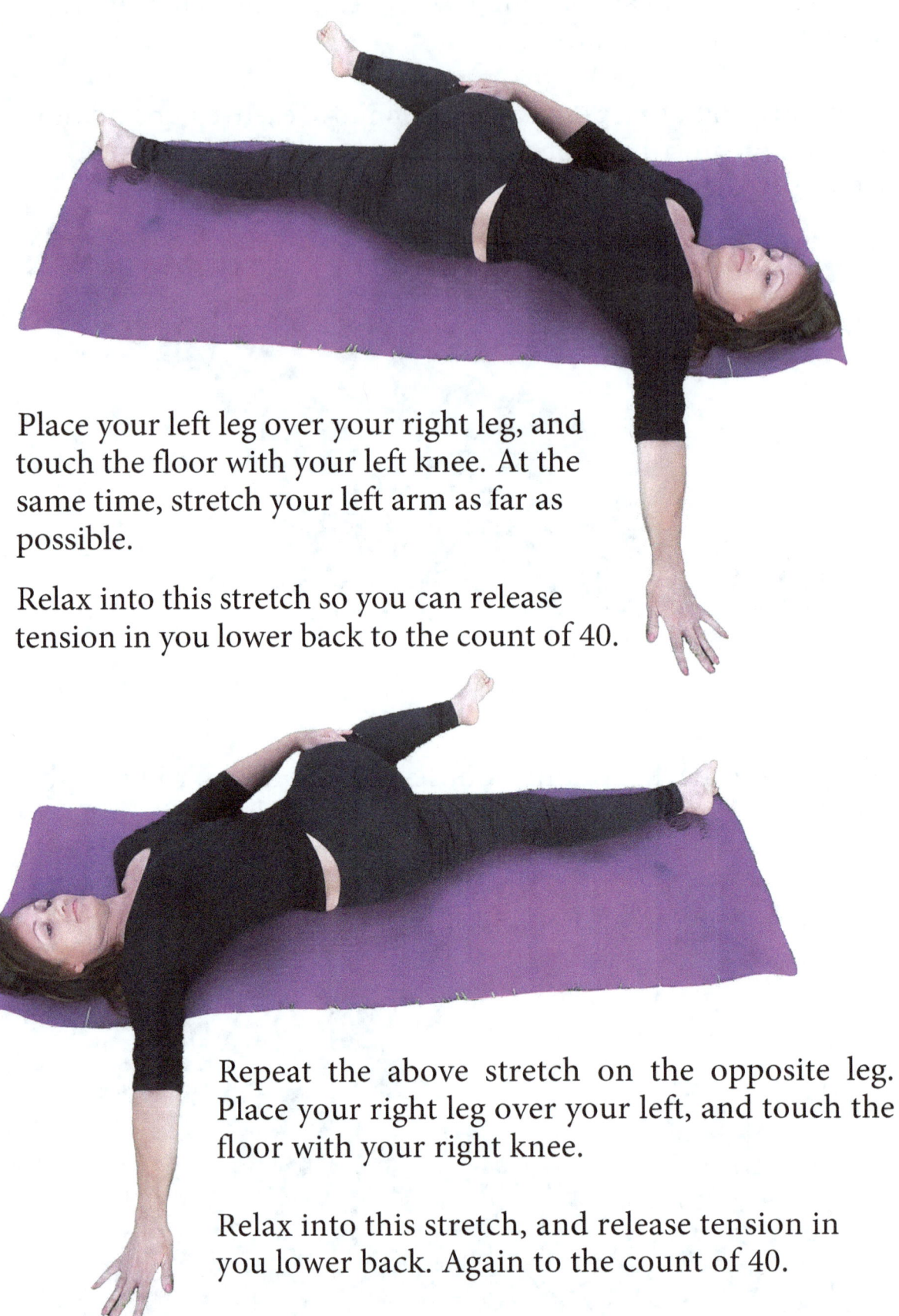

Place your left leg over your right leg, and touch the floor with your left knee. At the same time, stretch your left arm as far as possible.

Relax into this stretch so you can release tension in you lower back to the count of 40.

Repeat the above stretch on the opposite leg. Place your right leg over your left, and touch the floor with your right knee.

Relax into this stretch, and release tension in you lower back. Again to the count of 40.

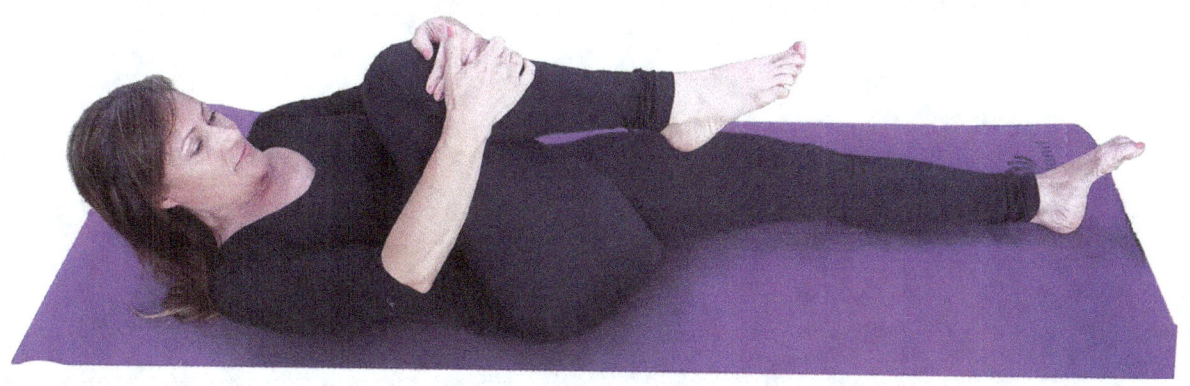

Hold your right knee up to your chest. Feel the stretch in your lower back. Repeat with your left knee. Then, crunch both left and right legs together into your chest. Do each 3 movements to the count of 20.

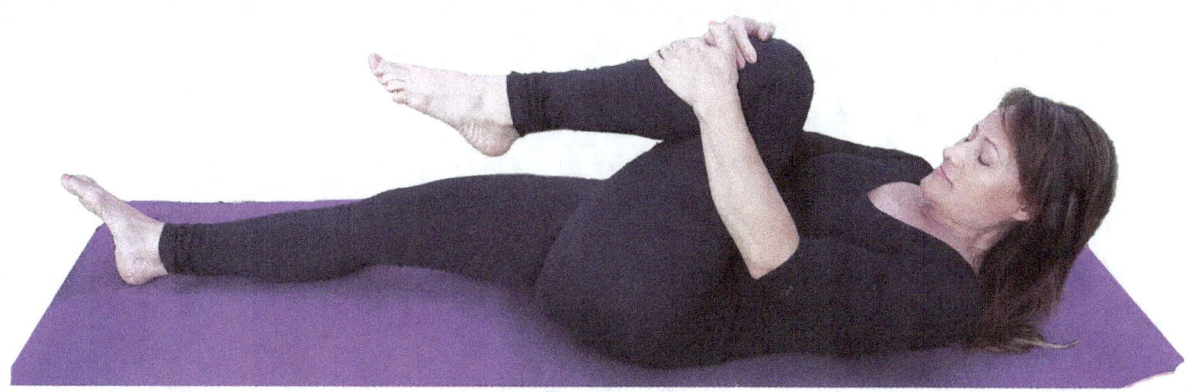

Finally, remain on your back and spread your arms and legs out "star shaped" as pictured on this workbook's cover. Take pleasure in feeling the flow of energy this routine stimulates throughout your body. Do this "Tune-Up" routine daily as it will harmonize the flow of energy, stimulate balance, and increase vitality throughout your day.

Through continued practice, you will promote health and vigor, while stimulating a sense of joy and eagerness for living life. Additionally, this practice will amplify your feeling of being in contact with your body, while massaging away aches and pains. Finally, you may experience welcoming synchronistic events as your inner spirit is now connecting with the energy flow that life provides.

Feel free to add any other movements or stretches to your routine that helps you feel more connected to this flow of energy within your body.

—Part 2—
Mind

The Brain vs. The Mind

There is a distinct difference between the Brain organ and the Mind. The Brain is the Central Processing Unit hardware of your body. Think of it as the CPU in your computer. It controls all of your automatic physical functions through the brain stem. It connects to every part of your body. It automatically functions to balance and regulate every aspect of this bio-energy being we call your body. It controls all your hormones, blood flow, heartbeat, and breathing. Everything! It requires no intervention or thought whatsoever.

The Brain also has multiple functions. Numerous physical regions within the Brain connect to the various sensory windows we call the senses. We commonly call the hearing, seeing, smelling, tasting, and feeling of the external world our sensors. These areas of the Brain include the front, sides and back of the Brain.

However, there is a sixth sense known as Proprioceptors. These neuro-sensors spread throughout every millimeter of your body providing a symphony of information unavailable to the 20% of the Broca's Area thinking portion of the Brain. This sixth sense is always available to you and provides the exact position of every part of your body.

The Mind is the software programmed into the Brain, which runs your internal and external awareness. The inner awareness we call "Yourself." Experiences are the software that programs the Mind. Think of it as a map or framework for navigating and interacting with your world. Essentially this software programs your conscience style on how you relate to yourself and life.

Thoughts shape your reality by creating a language framework of the world. For some, thoughts can constrict this framework creating a cage limiting the possibility to experience and understand oneself and the actual world. In truth, this inner sense of self is our programming and filters through our linguistic framework. Of course, this programming also creates our social experience.

Meditation 1

Find a comfortable sitting position. Sit with your back straight, not lounging. Hold your sitting as still as comfortable from 15 to 30 minutes. Allow your thoughts to   wander, remembering what your thoughts are saying to you. See if you can determine the themes your thoughts are suggesting. Usually the themes are three or four in total. If sitting becomes uncomfortable, you can lie on the floor, spreading your arms and legs apart as pictured in the front of this workbook.

At the end of the 15 to 30 minutes, write down all the thoughts you heard. Stay on this meditation until you have accomplished this step. Once mastered, move on to the next meditation.

Meditation 2

Again sit perfectly still as before. But now, work on inhibiting all thoughts of care, worry, and fear. Those are the thoughts you've probably heard echoing in your mind repetitively over time. They are the type of thoughts that take you nowhere, that won't lead you anywhere, thoughts that are simply a dead-end to nowhere.

Tell your mind "Thank you, I've heard those thoughts a thousand times! I got it! I don't need to hear you telling me those thoughts anymore."

Instead, allow only thoughts of what you'd like to achieve in life. Allow yourself to create and entertain only thoughts of what you desire to see unfold in your lifetime. Thoughts of what you'd like to build upon, thoughts of how you'd like to see your life moving forward and unfolding over time towards achievement.

You may only be able to do this for only a few moments at a time. After the exercise, write down what thoughts came to you, and what thoughts would potentially   build a future you'd like to enjoy in life. Stay on this meditation until you have accomplished this step. Once mastered, move on to the next meditation. Again, do this until you are clear and certain about what thoughts you'd like to build upon for your life.

Remember:
Thoughts are things that create your reality.

Meditation 3

Again sit perfectly still as before. Now attempt to inhibit all thoughts. This time concentrate on simply relaxing your muscles. Turn mindful attention to sensing your body. Allow all your muscles to return to a relaxed condition. Remove the pressure on your shoulders and allow your muscles to relax. Invite your body to completely relax and allow yourself to breathe deeply.

Concentrate on the feeling of your blood flowing in the form of energy circulating freely from your head to your toes. Use mindfulness to feel your body. The proprioceptors tell you what position every part of your body is in, so pay close attention to them.

Focus your attention to feel your skull from the inside. Then feel your entire head. Move to feel your face from the inside; then your ears; moving into your neck; then shoulders. Then focus your attention on your chest cavity. Feel how your chest expands and contracts with every breath you take. Now focus on the strength of your spine; then focus upon your back; move to feel your hips, then the pelvis, and then your butt. Moving on to your thighs, followed by your knees, calves, ankles, feet, and finally your toes. Feel how to contact your body and learn this method to love yourself.

Simply use your mind to navigate and dance up and down throughout your body, allowing a pleasurable inner dance that causes your entire body to relax. Allow yourself to contact a sense of energy flowing freely throughout your body.

Physical tensions produce mental unrest. Tensions cause heightened abnormal mental activity of worry, care, fear, and anxiety. Relaxing your body allows your mind to grow quiet and restful. It allows you to feel peaceful within yourself and feel peaceful in the world that surrounds you. Allow your stomach area to relax, release tension, and allow your entire physical being to imagine you are pressing light and energy outward into the world.

Thoughts are simply internal speech. When you think, your vocal cords slightly move as though you are speaking aloud. And your tongue will move ever so slightly forming your silent words.

One technique to help you quiet your mind is to "hold your tongue." Touch the tip of your tongue to where your front teeth meet the roof of your mouth. Hold your tongue still, and watch how you no longer think thoughts.

Stay on this meditation until you have accomplished this step. Once mastered, move on to the next meditation. Do this meditation until you have mastered the art of remaining internally silent.

Meditation 4

Take your usual seating position. Now navigate your mind to dance through your inner body toward relaxing all your tensions and muscles as before. Reactivate the feeling tone of allowing yourself to feel the flow of energy throughout your inner unified body. Press your imaginary energy outward into the world. Imagine you are saying none verbally, "I am pressing my physical energy outward, offering my energy outward, and opening to receive the life-giving energies of the world surrounding me. I choose to be energetically present, pressing my energy outward, open to receive life-promoting energy from this incredible life-producing planet. The world created me, and I'm an intrinsic part of all creation."

Choose to release all thoughts of worry, jealousy, envy, sorrow, anger, hatred, and disappointment of any and all kinds. Understand that negative thoughts do not lead you toward any fulfilling path. Negative thoughts only prevent you from moving forward toward embarking upon a path of your own creation, and only cause discomfort.

Just determine mentally to voluntarily release all of those negative thoughts. Refuse to entertain any negative thoughts that lead to perpetuating loss, sadness, disappointment, and self-incrimination. Recognize you are the one choosing to think these thoughts. Commit your mind from thinking any thoughts that take you away from any feeling connected to the joy of being your body, and move towards fulfilling your life.

Remember, all these negative, self-deprecating thoughts are only learned behaviors, forced upon you when you were young. In school, you were taught to sit still, stop focusing on your body, and just pay attention to the words spoken to you. You were taught this to stop you from feeling free and happy within your body. Instead, they taught you that time is a machine on a wall. That words and ideas are who you are. Your place is in society, and your job is to conform to the power of words and numbers.

Begin to learn how to contact your inner energy. Do this by utilizing your entire mind. Gain control over your thoughts by contacting the energy within your body. This is just a beginning. This process can awaken you that your body is actually alive with energy connected to life, but your "thoughts only create an imaginary reality."

Soon you will come to realize you have the power to choose to dismiss and release all negative and destructive thoughts. You will realize this because you'll see that negative thoughts fail to lead you toward creating the life you wish to lead. The only thoughts that lead you toward fulfilling your dreams, are the thoughts that open up a path toward creating the life you desire to manifest.

Stay on this meditation until you have accomplished this step. Once mastered, move on to the next meditation.

Meditation 5

Again sit perfectly still in your place. Take some time to relax your body as you did in the previous lessons. Now imagine a time and place that has pleasant associations for you. Think of a place where you were completely happy and felt complete and joyful.

Create a mental picture of this place. See the buildings, the grounds, the trees, your friends, and all associations to this event. Repeat this exercise as often as you wish, so you can make mental pictures of pleasant experiences. Stay on this meditation until you have accomplished this step. Once mastered, move on to the next meditation.

Meditation 6

Return to your seating position again. Navigate through your body as before. Bring a photograph you like. Spend about 10 minutes looking at all the details of the picture. Examine it closely. Note the expression on the eyes, the clothing, the feeling tone of the photograph. Take your time to note every possible detail of the photograph.

Now close your eyes. Go through your dance of relaxing your body. Now recreate the picture in your mind's eye. See every detail. Recreate the picture in your mind. This will increase your mental powers to direct your mind to pay attention and focus on exercising your own willpower.

Should you have trouble doing this exercise, reopen your eyes, restudy the picture, and again recreate it in your mind's eye. Stay on this meditation until you have accomplished this step. Once mastered, move on to the next meditation. Repeat this exercise until it is something you are fully capable of imagining.

Meditation 7

Sit in your special place. Relax your body as before. Now imagine a pleasant conversation with a friend. See the friend exactly as you last saw him or her. See the room. See his or her face, see it distinctly. Now talk with them about a subject of mutual interest. See their expressions change. See their smiles. Create a new conversation with them, and listen to what they have to say to you.

By doing this you are increasing your ability to imagine what you want to create in life. This is simply another step in creating the power you need to ultimately be yourself. Stay on this meditation until you have accomplished this step. Once mastered, move on to the next meditation.

Meditation 8

Learning to break mental habits. This can be done by learning to replace destructive thoughts with constructive thoughts. Destructive thoughts are any thoughts that lead to sadness, loss, and an unfulfilled destination. Whenever you have a thought that diminishes you or your life's goals, simply replace it with a thought that returns you to a path leading towards joy, happiness, and life's ultimate fulfillment.

In this way, you learn to stop destructive "wrong thinking." When you hear a thought that leads you to a place you do not want to go, simply say, "That is a wrong thought, I'm replacing it with a thought that will take me towards a path I want to go." Thus you are entering the process of learning how to rid yourself of any thoughts that do not lead toward your happiness, joy, and fulfillment. "Right Thinking" is any thought that makes you feel good, and puts you on a path toward creating the life you wish to create.

"Tell your mind this is a fruitless thought. You've heard it a thousand times before, it leads me nowhere! It's a dead end and does not lead me towards creating a happy and fulfilled life." Stay on this meditation until you have accomplished this step. Once mastered, move on to the next meditation.

Meditation 9

Sit in your place. Navigate through your body to relax your muscles from head to toe as before. Imagine you are pressing your energy into the world surrounding you. Imagine you are radiating your energy from the left and right sides of your body. At the same time open yourself to receive the life-affirming energies of Earth embracing you. Imagine that the life force of Earth is here guiding and nourishing your evolution to grow into your highest and best self.

Concentrate upon the concept of *Plugging In to the Energies of Now*. Tell yourself that your inner experience is connected to the outer environment's creative energies. Allow a sense of harmony and connectedness to press outward into the world. Imagine that this energetic harmony from within and without is flowing and enhancing your experience of being alive. Feel both outer and inner worlds melding into an oceanic feeling harmony both inside and outside of your body.

Relax again within your body from head to toe. Imagine you are pressing your energy into the environment that surrounds you. In a non-verbal fashion say, "I am pressing my energy into the world, in this present moment, communicating with the world that I am here and present. I am allowing myself to open to receive energies to nourish and contribute to my life experiences. I am allowing both outer and inner energy to become one. My sensations are connecting to the flow of being."

This is the psychological oceanic experience of entering the flow. It is the basis of experiencing the vital energy of being alive within your body and connecting to the higher forces of nature. Simply imagine you are pressing your energy outward into the world that surrounds you. At the same time open to Earth's life force that causes all living things to evolve into their highest and best forms. Say in a non-verbal way, "I'm pressing my energy outward, and open to receive life's nourishing synchronistic experiences." Stay on this meditation until you have accomplished this step. Once mastered, move on to the next meditation.

Meditation 10

Sit in your place. Navigate through your body to relax your muscles from head to toe as before. Imagine you are pressing your energy into the world surrounding you. Now concentrate on the concept of the word "Love." Focus upon your heart within your chest. Feel a growing warmth in your heart and chest. Allow this feeling to grow and allow this feeling to give you a sense of pleasure within your chest cavity.

Stay on this meditation until you have accomplished a sense of pleasure within your heart. Once mastered, move on to the last meditation.

Meditation 11

Sit in your place. Navigate through your body to relax your muscles from head to toe as before. Imagine you are pressing your energy into the world surrounding you, and open to the nourishing energies that Earth is generating for all living creations to evolve into their highest and best forms. Now concentrate on the concept of the word *"Abundance."* Imagine your sense of self to expand outward into the infinite with "abundance." Continue this meditation until you have increased your sense of pleasure now within your being.

Once you learn the feeling of experiencing these 11 Meditations, you will no longer need to sit in your place. You can choose to look inward, and press your energy outward any time you desire. In this conscience way, you are opening to receive the life force energy that is always available. Anytime, anywhere you can choose to enter the ever-pervasive flow of being in the NOW.

Should you you ever feel uncomfortable, simply imagine pressing your energy outward into the world surrounding you. Anytime things get ruff. Anytime you need life to start working for your benefit, do this simple meditation. You will relax your shoulders, neck, and breath easier. Enjoy choosing this natural state of relaxing your body.

This is a process of opening your awareness to using 100% of your mind. Every time you revisit this meditation, you will begin to experience amazing synchronistic events. The world will open its cornucopia of offerings to you, and propel you toward evolving into your highest and best self. Watch doors open, and lights turn green, as smiling happy people who already know this awareness in consciousness greet you with love and acknowledgment.

—Part 3—
Spirit

How to Reach Enlightenment

Enlightenment is a concept that means different things to different people, and there are many paths that people follow to try to achieve them. Some people believe that enlightenment is a state of inner peace and understanding, while others see it as a state of perfect awareness or a oneness with the universe. There are no specific steps that you can follow to reach enlightenment, as the journey is a personal one that is different for each individual. However, there are some common practices that people often follow on their path to enlightenment, including:

-Living in the present moment by practicing mindfulness.

-Exploring spiritual practices such as meditation, yoga, or prayer.

-Seeking wisdom and understanding through study and reflection.

-Cultivating positive qualities such as compassion, kindness, and forgiveness

-Letting go of attachments and ego-driven desires.

-It's important to remember that enlightenment is not a destination that you can reach, but rather a journey of continuous self-discovery and growth.

How to Become Spiritually Aware

There are many ways that people can work to become more spiritually aware. Some common practices include:

Meditation: Meditation can help you quiet your mind and connect with your inner self. Practicing mindfulness: Being mindful means connecting inward and paying attention to your breathing, thoughts, and feelings without judgment in the present moment.

Exploring different spiritual traditions: Reading about and learning about different spiritual traditions can help you gain a greater understanding of this world and the ongoing process of fitting in with it.

Engaging in prayer or spiritual rituals: Many people find that participating in prayer or spiritual rituals focuses their mind to feel more connected to a higher power of existing energy, creating a path of direction and purpose.

Seeking guidance from a spiritual teacher or mentor: Connecting with a spiritual teacher or mentor can provide you with guidance and support as you explore your inner spiritual beliefs.

Remember that becoming spiritually aware is a journeying process, and it will look different for everyone. Be open to exploring and discovering what works for you.

Why are We Here?

What is the purpose of the Universe? During a silent weekend meditation retreat, I blurted out during the silent meditation "What is the purpose of the Universe?" Surprisingly, the Buddhist monk meditation leader responded, "The purpose of the Universe is to express energy."

Here we are, living on the only planet in the Universe that has created us and supports our species. A world that is nourishing all living things to grow into their highest and best selves. Earth is evolving all these forms of life - in abundance and interconnectedness.

Humankind lives under one of its most incredible illusions - we believe we are somehow separate and apart from this miraculous and fantastic environment we call planet Earth. Those in power would have you think your true purpose is to be a good worker, to take orders from a superior, to be on clock time, and pay your taxes.

We are trained to sit at a desk, be still, be quiet, and restrain ourselves. Not to feel free to discover our true nature, but programmed to think and listen to ideas. We are programmed to see an alternative world of ideas in words. We've spent years and years learning words. Can you guess the number of words drilled into your mind? Anywhere from 10,000 to 40,000! You've been spoon-fed so many words that you've learned how to talk to yourself all the time. So many words creates a framework to look at life and how to think. You have a programmed way to experience your entire existence.

They trained you to have a framework to name everything of the outside world through symbolic sounds, which we call words and numbers. However, for some, this framework has become a cage that limits how we experience the world because it is filtered through this framework of learned thoughts.

We go through our lives constantly projecting our linguistic framework onto the world. This framework predetermines and filters everything we see and feel. While this is happening, we discuss our experiences incessantly to our selves with our thoughts. Many times this framework hampers us from seeing any new possibilities in our world. And sometimes, these thoughts won't stop thinking.

What are words and ideas? What is this predetermined framework that interprets our experience? Words are "sound symbols" for things, feelings, theories, and thoughts. We were taught to see these sound symbols within our minds. Words are not the actual objects of experience. They are only symbolic representations of actual things, experiences, feelings, and ideas.

Since words are only sound symbols of actuality, we've come to believe our thoughts are reality. However, they are not the ACTUAL EXPERIENCE of that which we are thinking! They are only an imaginative representation of actuality. They are not actuality!

The logical framework of language rests upon opposing forces called constructs. UP vs. Down. Good vs. Evil. Happy vs. Sad. Kind vs. Mean. Rich vs. Poor. They describe and build a mental framework that allows you to manipulate this symbolic world in fantasy. However, these thoughts are not the actual things we are thinking.

What's the problem here? Many of us believe our thoughts are reality and that the world is an "out of reach" illusion instead of the other way around. Many see themselves as separate, alone, and not part of this world we live in.

Instead of learning to employ all our senses and all our mind's capabilities, we have been trained only see our world through the language portion of our mind. The brain's thought region consists of only about 10% of your brain. By staying only within our thoughts, we fail to use the rest of the 90% of our brain's power. By relying solely on thought, we might fail to contact with the other parts of the brain that process vision, sounds, physical body senses, and the intuition that the combined integration of all our sensors creates.

The most significant detriment of viewing life only through our thoughts is we fail to grow, enhance, expand, and contact our inner sense of self and energy. There are no word symbols that can embrace our inner body experience. This socialization process created a framework through which we see and share our outer world reality. The inner world of personal intimacy can not be experienced verbally. You can point with symbols to it, but that is not the actual experience.

So why are we alive? Is it to be good citizens? To pay our taxes and be good students, or good workers for a corporation or superior? There must be more to life than that!

Perhaps the true purpose of this temporary gift of life is to develop a solid inner being fed by experience. Maybe life is a pilgrimage designed to produce a strong and lasting inner sense of self. Considering your body is the temple of your soul or spirit, our mission in this life might be to nurture and grow a powerful inner sense of self realization.

Eventually, our bodies will die and no longer support our inner sense of self. Perhaps we have been offered this miraculous gift of life to develop a higher level of awareness and connection to energy. As Einstein said, "Energy can not be created or destroyed; it can only change form." When your body can no longer support your inner being, maybe during the course of your lifetime, you have gathered enough spiritual energy to move forward into what might be the next level of conscientiousness.

Countless accounts of near-death experiences all point to something beyond this life we call living. People with near-death experiences consistently report a liberating feeling of freedom from the body. They report feeling pleasure, love, serenity, and liberation that is liken to joining a grater source of white light energy.

All cultures point to the existence of an afterlife. Some words include heaven, Valhalla, eternity, everlastingness, the hereafter, immortality, reincarnation, eternal, and allegory. The single word "soul" sums up that there is an essence of existence that transcends this worldly physical plane.

In many cultures, there is a belief that you can pray to your ancestors, that they still exist on a spiritual plane and can aid you in this life.

How do you cultivate a solid inner spiritual garden? How can you support, flourish, and enhance a sense of inner being? You can by simply gazing inward toward the heart region within your chest. By doing this, you can feel the energy of love in your heart. Your heart and chest area has more electro/magnetic energy than any other organ in your body. Yet no one has ever taught you to seek the answer within and "feel" something that's always been within you.

By applying a portion of your mental energy to look inward, you can cultivate a sense of an inner space that is yours and yours alone. Calling this introspection, you can periodically direct an aspect of your mind to connect with the feeling tone or vibration of energy flowing within your heart and your entire body.

This feeling tone has always been available to you. However, through conditioning, from an early age onward, thinking has replaced feeling the constant flow of energy both within your body and the nourishing powers of the outside world. This vital energy constantly offers you a sense of joy, pleasure, and connection to life's support and wonderment. Just remember when you were a child, when words didn't replace your joy of being. Tapping this energy is simply gazing inward and contacting the power of feeling your breathing of life force.

The linguistic programming of society is to think and relate using sound symbols. Excessive thoughts in the form of sound symbols distract you from contacting and processing your total sensory awareness of both inner and outer energies. Thinking thoughts do take you on an illusionary adventure via imagination. Excessive thinking causes you to lose contact with the actual inner proprioceptors within your body and distracts you from integrating the here-and-now energies available through your senses.

The trick is simple. As soon as you realize you've broken contact with your body's "feeling tone" by thinking some thoughts, gently return your mind's focus to feeling grounded and centered in your chest cavity again. Notice the sensations of moving your arms and legs. Feel how your shoulders relax, release tensions in your neck, realign your posture, and take a small sigh of relief that you've released thinking fantasies. You've again just switched your focus back to the actuality of feeling and being in contact with contacting your senses.

Yet there is still another step. It is to imagine pressing your psychic energy outward so that a pleasurable oceanic feeling can connect you with the surrounding environment. I call this "Plugging-In" to your body and the present. As you sense you're pressing this invisible electrical, magnetic, and spiritual energy outward from the left and right sides of your body, you can feel, in a non-verbal fashion, "I'm communicating to the world by pressing my energy outwards and opening myself to receive life's nourishing energy from the world that surrounding me.

Feel the following without words, "I'm pressing my sense of energy outwards into the environment surrounding me. I'm allowing my inner self to accept Earth's nourishing and supportive energy. Earth's energy is helping every living entity to evolve into its highest and best self. This energy will also aid me to grow into my highest and best self. I'm allowing my shoulders and neck to relax, I'm regaining contact with my breathing and my senses. I'm feeling alive and connecting to life force energy."

By directing a part of your mind to "feel and contact all your senses," you can tap 100% of your mind and contact your moment-to-moment experience. Simply focusing on the symphony of sensations of your body when walking is an act of connecting with the here and now. Think of this as an ongoing meditation that you keep reminding yourself to revisit from time to time.

Release all learned illusions that you are separate and alone. By imagining, you are pressing your energy outward you are opening a pathway to receive power inward. By doing this imaginary non-linguistic practice, you are "plugging into the here-and-now of Earth's energetic biosphere field." The more you do this simple meditation within your moment-to-moment awareness, the more natural this awareness will become and anchor you into the here-and-now flow of living within your life's adventures.

Once you've freed yourself of the illusion you are separate from the surrounding environment, you can open yourself to the joy and pleasure of being connected to your body and the world surrounding you. You can open yourself to nourishing events known as synchronicities, kismet, happenstance, or coincidence.

Coincidence and synchronicity events are signposts telling you that you are truly entering the spiritual path of being plugged into and connecting with this fantastic world that manifested you!

Remember: Use your mind to come to your senses. *Being* is simply connecting with the flow of energy.